Speaking of

Yoga

Speaking of

Yoga

Pandit Shambhu Nath

A Sterling Paperback

STERLING PAPERBACKS
An imprint of
Sterling Publishers (P) Ltd.
A-59, Okhla Industrial Area, Phase-II, New Delhi-110020
Tel : 26386165, 26387070 Fax : 91-11-26383788
E-mail: ghai@nde.vsnl.net.in
Website : www.sterlingpublishers.com

Speaking of : Yoga

ISBN 81-207-1794-5

Published by Sterling Publishers Pvt. Ltd., New Delhi-110020
Printed at Sai Early Learners, New Delhi-110020

DEDICATED

on his 91st Birthday

to

Venerable Shri Yogendraji, The Father of Yoga Renaissance, sitting at whose feet I heard words of wisdom which instilled into me right ideas and inspired me on life's sacred journey.

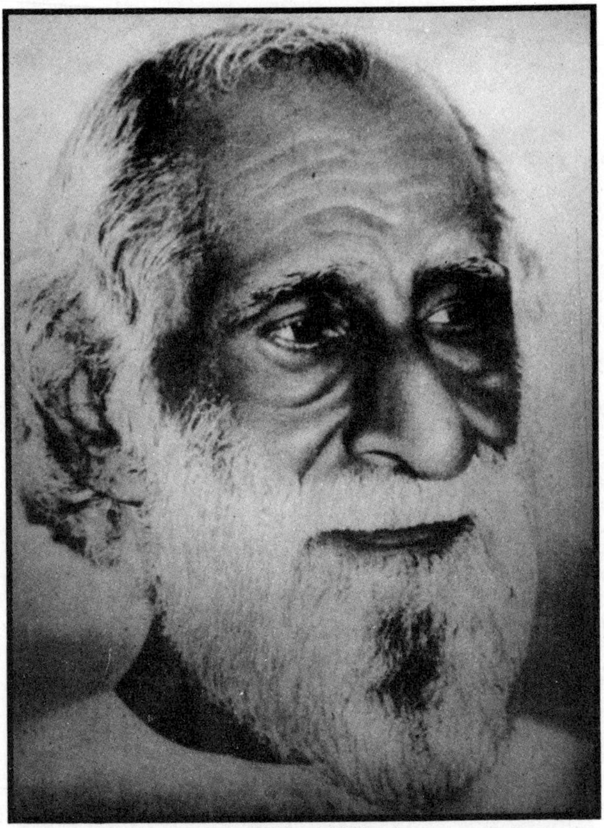

(1897 - 1989)
PIONEER OF SCIENTIFIC YOGA RENAISSANCE

"Yoga which studied man in depth at all levels has much to offer to project an alternative to the modern style of thinking and living. What is needed is to understand Yoga not as others understand it but as Patanjali understood and propagated it. In his classic system of Yoga, he has methodically shown what afflictions man suffers from and for what reasons. He has applied spiritual psychology to explore this and has supplied the basic technology for elevating man from his moorings of animal life. Those working for sublimation, integration and evolution of man will have no better alternative than the acceptance of Yoga as a way of life for future generations."

SHRI YOGENDRAJI

FOREWORD

Pandit Shambhu Nath is a fine product of The Yoga Institute, Santa Cruz, an institute that is devoted for the last 70 years to the popularisation of Yoga in a systematic and scientific way. Persons like Pandit Shambhu Nath who have been associated with The Yoga Institute on its staff for many years can be easily distinguished. Such persons are sincere and dedicated, and it takes just a little while to realize the difference between peddlers of spirituality and pseudo-yogins and genuine teachers of Yoga. When such a missionary teacher of Yoga decides to write a book on his experience of many years, the product becomes significant and intrinsically valuable. It matters little if Pandit Shambhu Nath is not a literary wizard so long as what he writes is useful to and understood by a busy executive, an overworked physician or a tensed-up artist or worker. I am sure this book will be found helpful to the intellectuals who are not acquainted with Yoga but who would like to read and practise something simple that can mean good health, mental tranquillity and spiritual poise.

Dr. Jayadeva Yogendra

ACKNOWLEDGEMENTS

I express my deep debt of gratitude to Dr. Jayadevaji Yogendra–the principal of the Yoga Academy of the Yoga Institute, Santa Cruz, Bombay, who not only taught me all that I know of Yoga but has been to me a friend, philosopher and guide.

I am also grateful to Mother Sita Devi but for whose guidance, encouragement, love and affection, I would not have ventured to write this book.

My special thanks are due to Shri Kamal Kumar for going through the manuscript and making valuable changes and necessary corrections, and also to Shri Y.K. Sharma of St. Stephen's College for his constructive discussion.

My gratitude to Cecilia and Sandeep Chandra who, after going through our 2-month Better Living Course, have posed for these photographs, and also to our Yoga Teacher Sheshpal Rastogi for his help in securing illustrations for the book.

My thanks also to Kitty Hazuria for the photographs included in the book.

ACKNOWLEDGEMENTS

PREFACE

The sophisticated industrial civilisation with its revolutionary and spectacular successes in the realms of the atom as well as outer space. is now faced with a value crisis. It witnesses a terrible disintegration of the human personality that results in abnormality, tension, anxiety, boredom and unhappiness in the society. In the most affluent societies of numerous developed countries too, today, material possessions and technology representing the ultimate value of life are proving themselves inadequate, nay, counter productive. Modern civilisation seems to promise everything except human happiness and peace. There seems to be much greater need today, if mankind is to survive, for the culture of the self which alone can ultimately ensure peace and happiness for the man. Without this, everything achieved materially or externally, as it were, will not only be far from being worthwhile but positively dangerous as well.

YOGA, the science of man–based on our ancient wisdom and culture–has laid down a technology consisting of various psycho-physio-logical processes for dealing with the body-mind complex. It tries to harmonise and integrate the human personality at all levels and stages of life. It shows the way out of the complexities and problems of life and holds the KEY TO BETTER LIVING.

The book presents the psychosomatic yoga technique for tackling all problems of both the mind and the body. It adopts a commonsense and rational approach in re-educating the modern man by giving him the basic guidelines to 'Better Living'. The short and long practical courses of 'Better Living' covering Twelve practices and Twenty-four practices at a time respectively, as a daily routine, have been worked out to give the maximum result in the minimum time through exercises which are not too vigorous or strenuous and are best suited both to the layman and the Sadhak (practitioner of Yoga) equally. These integrated courses have been carefully selected, well investigated and scientifically evaluated through half a century of research work carried out at the Yoga Institute of Santa Cruz Bombay–the pioneering institute dedicated to Yoga education, therapy and research in our country since 1918. These courses have been well tried at the institute and have been tested further by the author on thousands of students belonging to all age groups and from varying walks of life at New Delhi, with very encouraging results for the last fourteen years. One can initially take up the first basic "12 BL Course" and after developing a certain amount of flexibility of the spine thereby, one could graduate to the next graded "24 BL Course". Even the first basic course collectively gives one a feeling of freshness, more energy, physical tranquillity and mental peace, besides toning up the body system, solving minor health problems and redressing stress condition. To create in the Yoga aspirant a better understanding and greater appreciation of the subject in its true spirit, each element of Yoga technology is well explained first, followed by practicals under that category–graded from simple to moderately hard ones.

Special features of therapeutic asanas are mentioned with their manifold benefits that accrue when we ideally coordinate breathing rhythm with physical movement to derive maximum hygienic advantage from each asana. Economy of time is the principle observed in the selection of these asanas and only the essential ones are covered. Prime importance, however, is given to maintaining the structural integrity of human organism both in health and disease, with the cooperation of the nervous system. Standardised techniques of simple pranayama (breathing process) are included and so also certain yogic hygienic processes made safe enough for the common man. Special psychosomatic practices have been very much emphasized, to learn the art of neuromuscular relaxation and for quietude and stillness of the mind. The aim is that physical-cum-health education must effect the whole person (body-mind-complex) leading to self-control, concentration and mental purity (Chitta Shuddhi). The importance of diet reform from yogic as well as commonsense point of view is covered in recommending a health-promoting, vegetarian, well-balanced diet.

A separate section deals with guidelines on living through the techniques and principles available in Yoga, especially to help the modern man or woman who suffers much too much from psychosomatic problems. These techniques help in promoting greater self-awareness and understanding of self through motivations, value judgement, attitude and behaviour, which lead to a gradual change in one's HABITUAL REACTION PATTERN and better control of one's personality. With the help of psychosomatic and pranayama practices and by conditioning the mind and the body, one develops mental poise, serenity and ability to relax at will. All this and much more for self improvement is contained in the book, to enable an individual to become less inhibited and more and more integrated to lead a TENSION-FREE LIFE. It is the Yoga way of life, which, if practised daily, can make our life healthy, efficient, more creative and meaningful. This book will be of special interest and use to Yoga teachers as an aid who want to follow a classroom method of teaching, while being equally useful to the layman and uninitiated.

However, it should be remembered that the requisites for a safe and fruitful study of Yoga are:

...Strong motivation in personal development.

...Regularity of practice.

...Integral conditioning of the body-mind complex, and

...Implicit faith in nature which is infallible.

It is the Yoga way of life, which, if practised daily, with an attitude of detachment and devotion, alone can give a true INNER YOGIC EXPERIENCE and promote a built-in FAITH in one's inner self.

Shambhu Nath

CONTENTS

PART I

1

UNDERSTANDING OF YOGA

1.1 YOGA: POPULAR ILLUSIONS AND WRONG NOTIONS

Yoga has been for much too long construed as something connected with magic and miracles or with miraculous feats or endurance like being buried alive, flying in the air, walking on water or walking on burning coal, drinking acid, chewing glass, etc.

Quite a few still think that it is a system of stunts, gymnastic skills and of limb-twisting. To most of the rest yoga is a form of physical education whereby one has to attain proficiency in a few difficult asanas, gain mastery over a few spectacular kriyas and hold the breath in some form of kumbhak (or retention) for as long as possible. Many among those who claim to know about therapeutical value of yoga, believe that there are specifics for each disease in yoga and that what the yogin has to do is merely to describe some special asanas or breathing exercises or kriyas for various ailments.

If it is not understood at the physical level, it is understood by the masses as transcendental or instantaneous meditation, a modern craze prevalent in the West. To many, yoga also appears to be a technique of mystic experience only.

These are some of the common popular notions about the subject of yoga, emanating out of misinformation or ignorance.

Despite the wide publicity and propaganda about yoga in numerous countries of the world and the widespread adoption of its techniques by the medical, educational, social, cultural and spiritual institutions and organizations, the real yoga has still been clouded with various misconceptions and the average man remains confused about the aim and usefulness of yoga–the SCIENCE OF MAN.

1.2 WHAT YOGA MEANS

1.2.1 Philosophical and Traditional Meaning

VEDANTA: If the word is derived from the root YUJIR YOGE, it means 'to unite', to bind together, or 'to yoke'. It literally means 'union'. Here it is used to mean the union of the individual spirit (jivatman) with the Universal Spirit (paramatman). If it is derived from the root YUJ SAMADHAU, it means concentration or meditation.

BHAGAWAD GITA: The three main paths of Yoga are described as Yoga of Action, Yoga of Devotion and Yoga of Knowledge.

There are many brief definitions of yoga such as:

"Yoga is dexterity in action"–(Yoga karmasu kausalam) II-50.

"Evenness of mind is called yoga"–(Samatvam yoga ucyate) II-48.

"Severance from the union with pain is yoga" (dukh asamyogam viogam) VI-23.

PATANJALI: "Yoga is defined by Patanjali as the cessation of the modifications of chitta" (Yogah chitta vrittinirodhah). This cessation is brought about through 'concentration' or 'meditation' which is called 'yogah samadhih'.

1.2.2 As a Science

Yoga is the process of conscious evolution and realization. According to Shri Yogendraji, Founder/President of the Yoga Institute, Santa Cruz, Bombay: "Yoga represents the efforts, the path, the progress and the end of human evolution."

Yoga is a process of conscious unfolding of oneself whereby the physical, mental and spiritual nature of the individual attains its perfect development–the totality of the whole life. Yoga is a process of realisation, not merely confined to knowledge, where you see the reality face to face and after which there remains no doubt, no fear, no misery.

1.2.3 Yoga in Modern Life

Yoga is for pranimatra, i.e., for all created beings. It is in no way limited by race, age, sex, religion or creed. It is based on a deep understanding of man and his place in this world. All can take advantage of it and can see the direct result, benefits and joy which it can give to them in their daily life.

What is expected of yoga in modern life is beautifully expressed by Shri Yogendraji, "What the society expects from yoga today is physical health–what they term fitness–for efficiency, besides mental balance and quietude (Samatvam). They also expect emotional control so that man may not suffer from strain and tension causing psychosomatic ailments which are on the increase. And finally yoga should provide for contentment, happiness and peace within oneself."

1.3 THE SYSTEM AND ITS METHODOLOGY

1.3.1 Historical Perspective

Yoga based as it is, on our ancient wisdom and culture, is more than 5000 years old and has been referred to by two specific words. One is SANATAN which means eternal as the process of evolution. The very concept of evolution originated and developed with (Samkhya) yoga. It is a process of self-culture, self-evolution and self-realization. The other word used for yoga is PURATANA–(used in Bhagawad Gita–means very ancient. The source of yoga is found in the ancient Vedas, the Upanishads, the Gita and the Sutras of Patanjali.

In the past men were interested not so much in material objects but quest led them to go beyond matter. A certain part of their life was spent in understanding the issues and problems relating to the Universe, Man and the Spirit–in the search for the ultimate knowledge. In the very early period they used to do 'tapa', inflicting sufferings on themselves; probably they believed that when flesh suffered, the power of the soul rose. A man who suffered penance and austerity was considered to be a yogi, since he tried to prove himself superior to nature. There is mention of Mad Munis (in Rig Veda) standing on one leg and the leg withering away. Buddha, whose date of birth is fixed at about 560 B.C. in his discourses reveals the existence of yoga techniques. He speaks of coming across ascetics mortifying themselves and Tapasavin with their legs withered away. There were various irrelevant types of yoga technologies and methods in vogue. Buddha, of course, discarded all this and created a new path–Buddhist yoga, based on meditation and moral life. At some point of time the cult of supernatural powers started getting mixed up with yoga. Brahmachari–the unmarried man–who never settled down as a householder and who severed his relations with the society, came to be called a yogi. 'Charya' means in search of and 'Brahma' means Self (spiritual). Probably, at that time, those who were in search of 'Brahma' led a life of celibacy. Like that yoga went on acquiring different connotations and forms and in course of time some components were identified for yoga technology. In Maitrayani Upanishad, there is a mention of six-fold yoga leading to contemplation and absorption (samadhi). Thus Tapa, Penance, Austerity, Supernatural power, Brahmacharya and Dhyana became yoga. But all this gave to yoga a rigorous appearance and confusion still remained as to what yoga actually was.

1.3.2 Classic Yoga

It was Rishi Patanjali, rightly called the Father of Yoga, who around 200 b.c., compiled, synthesised, modified, systematised and refined yoga in a metaphysical whole, grafted on Samkhya philosophy and laid down eight steps which form the basis on which the whole system of yoga works. It was indeed the first classical attempt to interpret the subject. The eight steps consist of Yama, Niyama, Asana, Pranayama, Pratyahara, Dharna, Dhyana and Samadhi. These steps in perfect order, as they are, were formulated on the basis of psychological understanding of the human mind. Yoga had recognised and accepted the importance of the mind and the subconscious over the total human personality much earlier than did the modern psychology in its present form. In the methodology of Pantanjali all the eight limbs or constituents are to be present in the same sequence with their correlation and ratios as recommended, to make the process of yoga successful. Yoga, thus, is a step-wise, stagewise eight-fold path to final liberation from pain and suffering. These steps progressively take you to the highest state of creativity, of discriminative knowledge and towards attaining the desired perfection. There lies its great purpose and usefulness. There are some who emphasise on only one or the other aspects of yoga, missing the integrated approach which is so classic and can alone give a total education for the transformation of the human personality from the disintegrated into an integrated one, sublimate man to divinity (from the ignoble to the noble is yoga). The classic yoga, commonly known as the eight-fold path (ashtanga yoga), covers both the yoga ideology and technology. The eight steps are:

YAMA	– Conditioned yoga behaviour, both personal and social.
NIYAMA	– Attitude sublimated to yoga norms.
ASANA	– Discipline of the physical body.

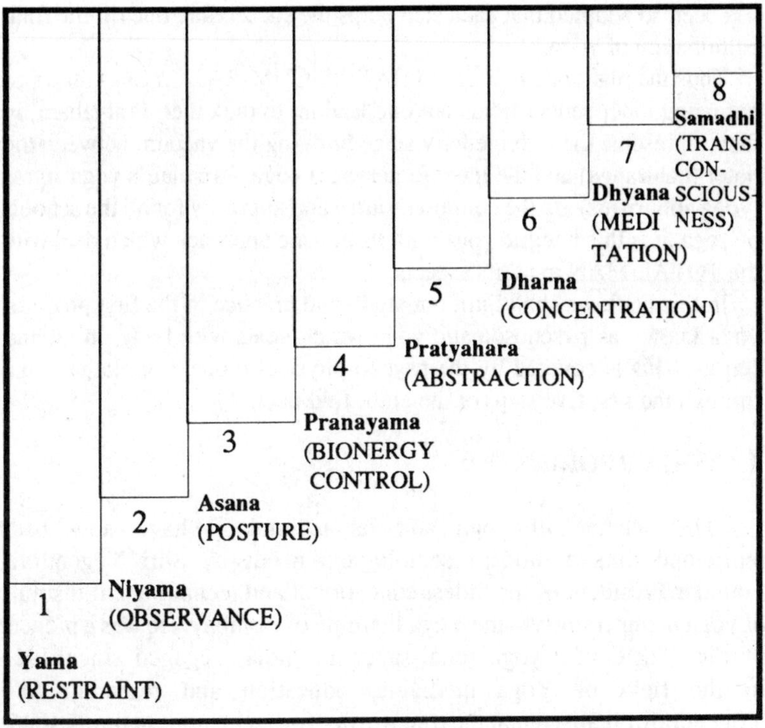

PRANAYAMA	– Control over bioenergy through respiratory action.
PRATYAHARA	– Withdrawal of the senses inwards through abstraction.
DHARNA	– Concentration.
DHYANA	– Meditation
SAMADHI	– Consciousness absolute or transconsciousness (KAIVALYA)

Of these, the first five which border on the PSYCHOSOMATIC APPROACH are referred to as External (Bahiranga) yoga, popularly known as HATHA YOGA, while the latter three which directly affect the psyche are known as Internal (Antaranga) yoga, popularly known as RAJA YOGA. It is almost impossible to try internal yoga (Raja Yoga) for the average man before accomplishing the external one (Hatha Yoga). The respective sequence of the eight steps as the standard methodology of yoga, has been so adopted that each step helps the succeeding one till the final culmination of yoga.

Thus the real yoga belongs to HATHA-CUM-RAJA YOGA, the two not being independent fields but one leading to the other. Pratyahara, in fact, represents the intermediary stage bridging the vacuum between the outer (bahiranga) and the inner (antaranga) yoga. Patanjali's yoga sutras (yoga aphorisms) are the common source and authority for all the schools of yoga. it is this integral yoga with its holistic approach which deal with the TOTAL MAN in all its aspects.

In this book we shall limit our study and practice to the first phase of yoga known as pyschosomatic yoga which deals with body, mind and senses. This is covered by the psycho-physical process of Hatha Yoga through the first five steps of the eight-fold path.

1.4 YOGA REORIENTED

The scheme of yoga and its technology have now been reoriented to suit modern sociological needs by Shri Yogendraji, Founder/President of the oldest educational and technological institute of yoga in our country—the Yoga Institute of Bombay. He was a pioneer of the scientific yoga renaissance in India, engaged since 1918 in the field of Yoga medicine, education and research. Shri Yogendraji, realised that the true worth of yoga in modern times, if it is to play its larger role today, is in the reintegration and restructure of man's personality. According to him, yoga is primarily an education not only of the conscious but also the subconscious mind. Its holistic approach can give a TOTAL EDUCATION OF THE WHOLE MAN, harmonizing and reintegrating the individual personality at all levels of consciousness–physical, mental, moral, intellectual, emotional and spiritual and thus it fills the gap left by modern system of education. By simplifying the practices of yoga he has made it possible for the common man to achieve a better, fuller and richer life without undergoing the rigours normally associated with the traditional yoga.

An educational programme of yoga has thus been evolved based on classic yoga techniques with variegated elements of yoga technology. The practical Better Living Courses covered in the book consists of five distinct elements:

1. MENTAL CONDITIONING through meditative postures for better application of mind.

2. THERAPEUTIC ASANAS–careful selection has been made of asanas, especially for the spine and the abdomen, the two most important areas from the health point of view.
3. INTERNAL PURIFICATORY PROCESSES–made safe and easy.
4. SIMPLIFIED YOGENDRA PRANAYAMAS for an all-round benefit which not only help develop the respiratory system but also bring a tranquillizing effect on the mind.
5. SPECIAL PSYCHOSOMATIC PRACTICES for Neuromuscular relaxation and for quietening the mind.

These simple physiological and psychological processes of yoga collectively are useful for the health of the body-mind complex.

1.5 A PSYCHOSOMATIC APPROACH TO YOGA

In spite of all the amazing progress of science and technology, it is now being realised gradually by the great thinkers of the world in general and those of the West in particular that man's problems have multiplied several-fold. This has resulted in abnormality, tension, anxiety, boredom and unhappiness. Apart from organic, toxic-infective conditions and cases of injury, the treatment offered by the medical profession has failed to relieve human misery and suffering. The fact is widely accepted that at least seventy-two per cent of diseases today are psychosomatic diseases or stress diseases. This is the percentage in United States, the most affluent country in the world, according to Dr. Elmer Green, an American medical scientist.

'Psyche' is a Greek word meaning mind and 'soma' means the body. So psychosomatic diseases are those diseases which, while they have their origin in the psyche, are clinically diagnosed through somatic symptoms manifested in the body. In simple words it is all due to 'mind-body' problems, which have simultaneous interaction and mutual influence. Generally, it is believed that it is the emotional effects, caused by the stress and tension of modern life which are translated into somatic disorders. Ulcers, nervous and heart conditions, migraine, headache, asthma, colitis, eczema, diabetes, disorders of the digestive system, etc., are among the common psychosomatic complaints.

In yoga, diseases are of three types–(i) Bhautika or physiological (ii) Adhi Bhautika or psychological and (iii) Adhyatmika or psychic. But all these are interrelated–a fact which is hardly understood or appreciated by the modern physician. Yoga ideology admits that man lives not compartmentally, but at various levels–physical, mental, moral and spiritual–simultaneously. Basically, we have to understand that ill-health means some disharmony in the living organism. The homeostat mechanism is disturbed, a mechanism which has to be kept like a balance. The upsetting of the functional integrity of the body is expressed in many somatic symptoms. From the cause to the symptoms, there is a long chain of mis-alignment, maladjustment and malfunctioning, in the various interrelated components (koshas) of the body, causing disharmony (vighna). All these have to be adjusted to the point of integrated harmony like the tuning of a radio set. Instant relief or symptomatic relief therefore has no meaning, since yoga thinks that the process of nature takes its own time to re-establish the homeostasis normalcy. "If the causative factors persist which affect metabolism adversely, the disease will appear again or elsewhere and this pathogenic condition will continue till the yogic process of purification and unification is applied and the new yogic way of life accepted and followed."

Says Shri Yogendraji, "Yoga suggests an integrated approach to man with the personality-complex (chitta) as the basic factor and treats man as a body-mind complex."

Yoga was the first system in the world to recognize the connection and the interaction between the body and the mind. It has laid down psychosomatic means through its various psycho-physiological processes for dealing with the body-mind complex and tries to harmonise and integrate, the human personality at all levels and stages of life.

Integral conditioning of the body-mind complex through yamas will build up constructive, healthy, mental habits and attitudes with less ego involvement and attachment. A suitable course of postural training (asanas) of the exercises which are not too vigorous or strenuous, yoga hygienic process (kriyas), deep breathing methods (pranayama) and dietetics, all collectively make a positive contribution to perfectly harmonious health and fitness programme for an entire lifetime without recourse to medicines or drugs. Besides, under proper guidance, yoga holds that physical education should benefit the whole person and that the activities of asana and pranayama should be so conducted as to lead to self-control, concentration and mental purity (chitta-shuddhi).

Yoga techniques of the psychosomatic type will eventually bring about a state of neuro-muscular relaxation and increase the energy-level, thereby leading to mental poise and emotional stability. All yogic techniques are meant to provide a way of life and constitute an education in better or integrated living.

1.6 WHAT YOGA CAN DO FOR YOU

GOOD HEALTH, PREVENTION AND CURE OF DISEASE, SHARP ALERT MIND with increased powerof concentration for efficiency and precision.

ABILITY TO RELAX, to invigorate yourself mentally and physically if you are tired.

EMOTIONAL CONTROL results in POISE, FORTITUDE and EQUANIMITY by elimination of all problems of TENSION which lead to STRESS CONDITION.

PART II

2

LEARNING YOGA PRACTICES

It is obvious that a study of yoga is very different from that of any other subject such as history, geography or mathematics. It also does not deal with metaphysical speculation or philosophical discussion to satisfy your intellectual curiosity. It is the science of man and is, therefore, entirely concerned with the application of its technology in your daily life. The simple yogic techniques for health and self-improvement in this BL Course set out will benefit all. It is best to be taken as an experiment that you conduct on yourself, by yourself, for yourself. The three requisites for a fruitful study of the subject are:

Regularity of practice (abhyas),

Integral conditioning of the body-mind complex, a form of mental training and discipline, and

Implicit faith in Nature which is infallible.

2.1 HOW TO BEGIN

In any systematic study of yoga, a certain amount of preparation is definitely needed and so it is when you follow this integral course.

One of the objectives to be achieved in this course is to quieten the mind. Most of the time the mind is not at rest. It wanders a lot and is easily distracted. There may be conflicting ideas or thoughts or you may be emotionally upset. To get rid of all this agitation of the mind, you have to make an attempt to compose the mind through a process of conditioning. A proper mood thereby is created by way of inwardness, your mind too is quietened down and you are more receptive. You have the right frame of mind for any activity that follows. This conditioning is best achieved by sitting in a meditative pose. The adjustment of the posture with the lower extremities providing the fixity of the base, the trunk made straight with the spine erect, sitting motionless–all these are contributory factors to bring about the desired psychological and physiological results. Besides, it develops greater awareness and understanding of your body-mind relationship.

The central concept of learning meditative postures is to see whether we can withdraw our attention from the outside world and localise it on our body and its subtle working. It leads toa deeper awareness of one's body-mind complex. It is the first positive step to develop a subjective process of INWARDNESS.

2.2 MEDITATIVE POSTURES FOR CONDITIONING THE MIND

Sukhasana, while conforming to all these requirements, is the easiest asana to practise for a beginner. The very name indicates 'ease' and therefore steadiness. People who are used to sitting on chairs may have difficulty in the initial stages but for all others it is one of the easiest postures to adopt and practise. If you find difficulty in maintaining the spine erect, take the support of wall for your back.

THE INSTRUCTIONS

During the practice, the attention should shift from different parts of the body–head and neck; keeping the spine erect; keeping the abdomen drawn in a little and not allowing it to relax or possibly protrude; keeping the arms relaxed with no tension at elbow joints; shoulders drawn little backward; palms on knees. After keeping the mind busy for sometime in this way, one should bring one's attention slowly on breathing and simply watch passively one's own breathing rhythm without interference.

APPLICATION

For elimination of nervous agitation, composure, ease, breathing, conditioning, concentration.

Practise before starting your daily yoga routine practice or any activity.

2.2.1 Sukhasana (The Easy Pose)

(i) POSTURE: To sit in a crosslegged position with heels below the thigh and maintaining spine erect–Fig. 1 male).

(ii) METHOD

1. Sit with legs crossed at ankle.
2. Place heels comfortably below thighs.
3. Place palms on knees, elbows relaxed.

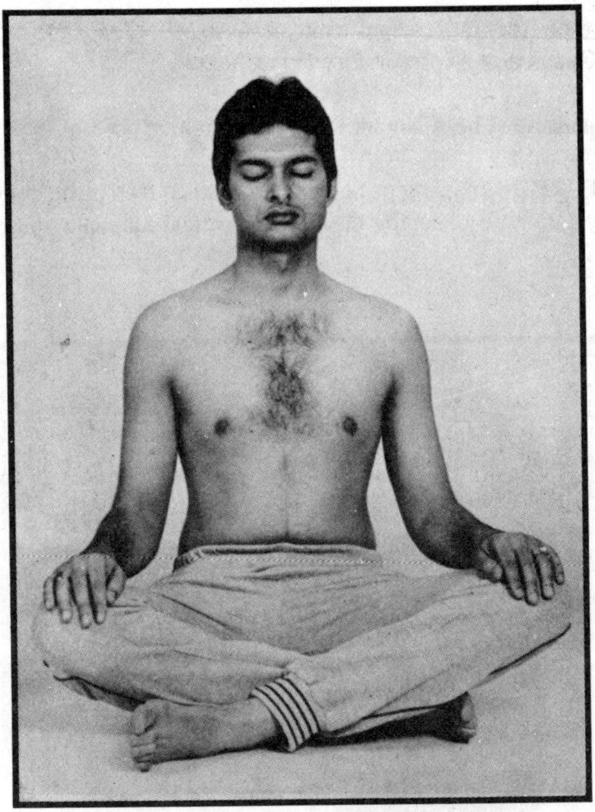

4. Maintain spine erect, head and neck straight.
5. Draw abdomen in normal contour.
6. Close eyes and mentally go through earlier instructions
7. Normal breathing.
8. Tell yourself to be quiet repeatedly as and when other thoughts try to come in.

(iii) RHYTHM: Normal breathing

(iv) DURATION: 7/10 minutes.

(v) BENEFITS: Corrects postural defects; loosens lower joints; provides fixity of base; promotes favourable circulatory changes –also in respiratory rate and pulse rate; leads to MENTAL CONDITIONING; and acts as preparatory to meditation.

2.2.2 Vajrasana (The Adamant Pose) A meditative posture

(i) POSTURE: In kneeling position with upturned feet, place buttocks in cavity formed by keeping the heels apart and maintain spine erect. (Fig. 2).

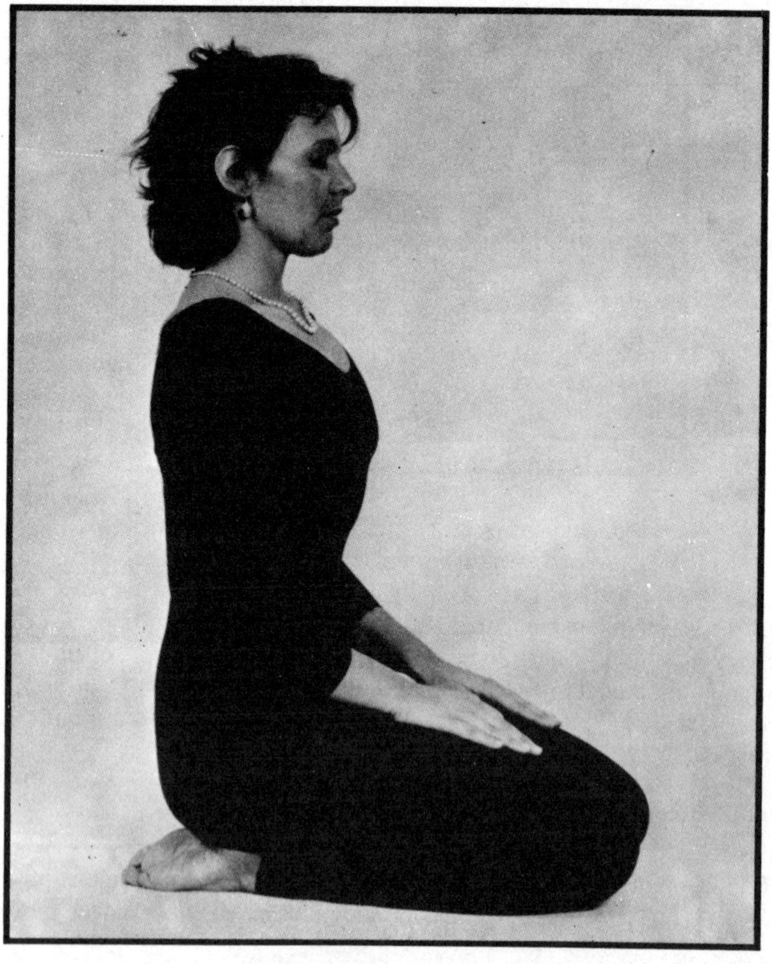

(ii) METHOD

1. Sit kneeling.
2. Slip toes to join at back, heels apart and the big toes pointed towards each other.
3. Place buttocks in cavity thus formed, thighs together.
4. Adjust hands on respective thighs, spine erect, head and neck straight.
5. Draw abdomen in contour.
6. Close eyes and mentally go through earlier instruc tions.
7. Watch normal breathing.
8. Tell yourself to be quiet repeatedly as and when other thoughts come in.

Note: If there is pain at the ankles or feeling of discomfort beyond your endurance (usual in the early stages of practice), use a soft cushion or fold your towel under your feet. Gradually increase the duration of practice from 3 minutes to 10 minutes. The great advantage of Vajrasana is that the spine is erect and is in a very correct position automatically. The ankle-joints stiffness and pain will disappear after practising for a week or so.

(iii) RHYTHM: Normal breathing.

(iv) DURATION: 5/7 minutes.

(v) BENEFITS: Corrects posture; better flexion of ankle and feet; relaxation of thigh muscle; good fixity; helps digestion and breathing; gives relief in backache; mental conditioning; preparatory step to meditation.

2.2.3 Padmasana (Lotus Pose) The classic meditative posture

(i) POSTURE: Folding the legs in a manner where soles of both the feet are turned up like the petals of a lotus flower, straighten your spine.

(ii) METHOD:

1. Sit with legs stretched forward.
2. Fold one leg (whichever is convenient), place the foot on the opposite thigh, heel pressing the pubic bone.
3. Similarly, bend the other leg in a way that the ankles cross each

other. In this way, each foot is on the opposite thigh with the soles turned upwards – the two heel ends almost touching each other– knees pressed to the ground (Fig. 3)

4. Rest palm on respective knee.
5. Keep the spine erect and neck straight as in Sukhasana.
6. Place left hand with its back touching the two heels– place the right hand overlapping on this. Keep eyes fixed on any object in front or keep eyes closed or gaze at the tip of the nose for concentration.

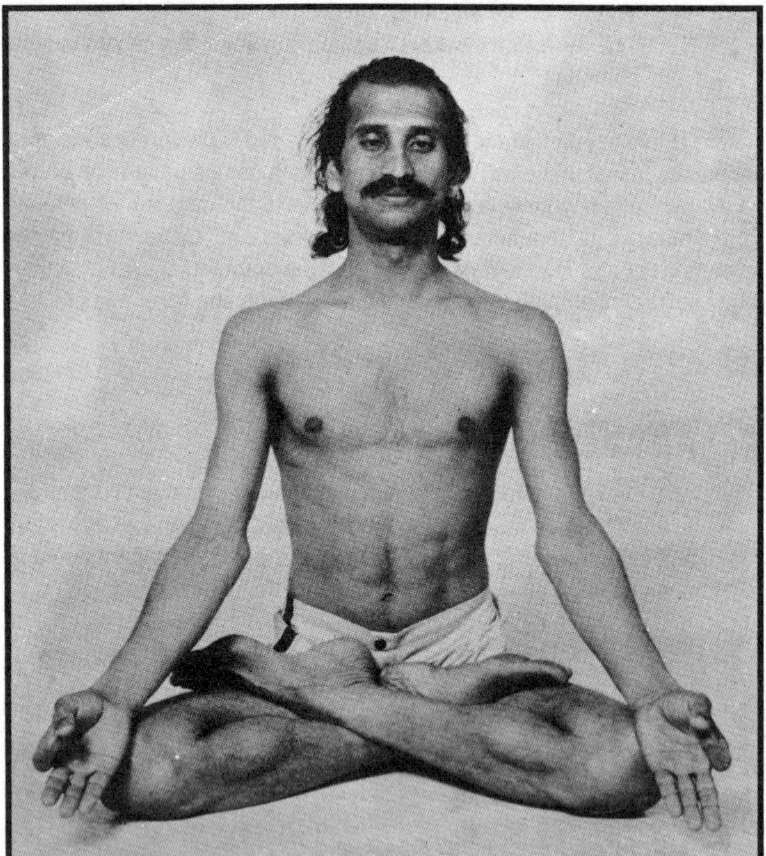

Initial problem: Heels not in level or knees not touching floor –persist on, with practice this can be corrected. If very difficult –first make an attempt with one foot upturned on the opposite thigh –interchange with the other foot.

(iii) RHYTHM: Normal breathing.

(iv) DURATION: 10 minutes.

(v) BENEFITS: Maximum fixity of base; corrective posture; preserves normal elasticity and especially helps all the important muscles, ligaments and tendons of the lower extremities; increases blood circulation in the abdomen-genital region; tones up the coccygeal and sacral regions of the spine and good for the sciatic nerve; better control over the seven principal chakras (lotuses); relieves constipation; recommended for practice of Pranayama, concentration and meditation.

Note:People suffering from low blood pressure should not perform this asana for a long duration.

2.2.4 Gomukhasana (Cow-Head Pose)

(i) POSTURE: Try to clasp the fingers of both hands behind shoulder blades, sitting with both legs bent in a manner where knees are overlapping (Fig. 4a).

(ii) METHOD: (For simple Gomukhasana)

1. Sit on the ground, fold left leg and keep the heel under the right buttock near the anus.
2. Fold the right leg over the left leg and bring the heel under the left hip as much as possible.
3. Keep both hands relaxed on the knees.
4. Keep the body straight, abdomen under control and spine erect.
5. Close your eyes and watch the breathing rhythm or gaze at the tip of the nose.

(iii) RHYTHM: Normal breathing.

(iv) COMPLETE GOMUKHASANA

6. Bring right arm up over the shoulder with the elbow bent in contact with your head (Fig. 4b).
7. Bring the other arm behind your back with elbow under your shoulder and upwards.
8. Try to clasp the fingers of both hands behind your back.

9. Close your eyes and keep normal breathing.
10. Alternate the position of the two arms along with the legs.

(v) BENEFITS: Improves circulation in and around armpits and the-sides; tones up the muscles, tendons and ligaments of the knees; relieves backache; favourable improvement in circulation and activity of both the lungs.

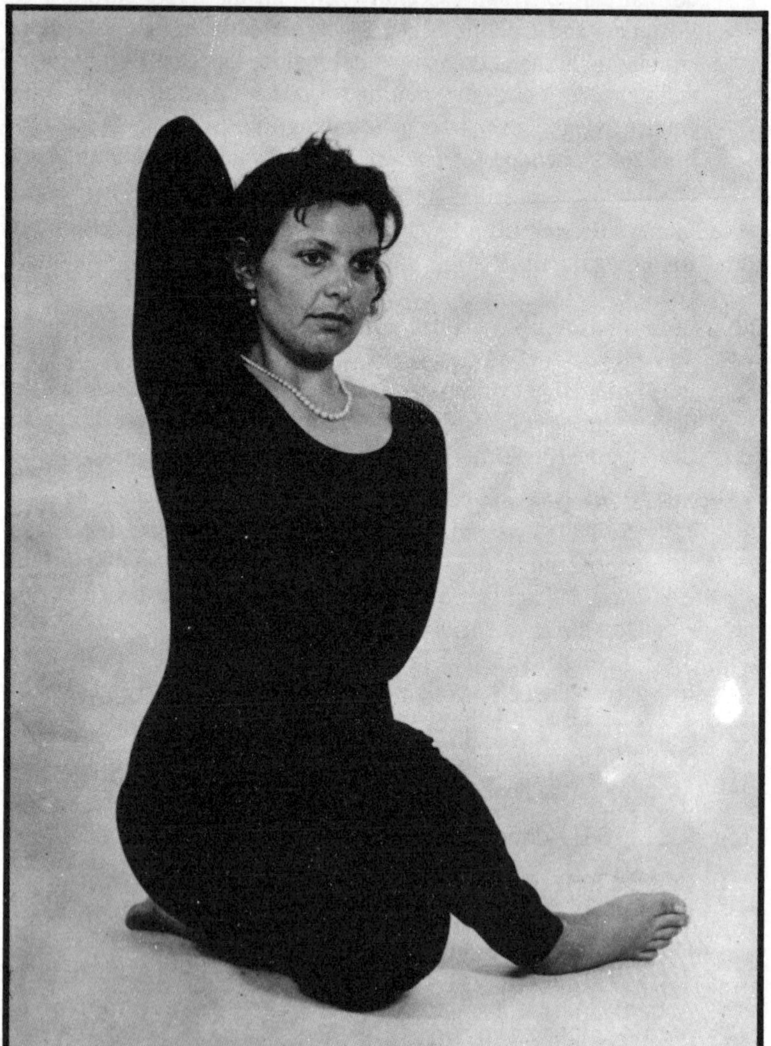

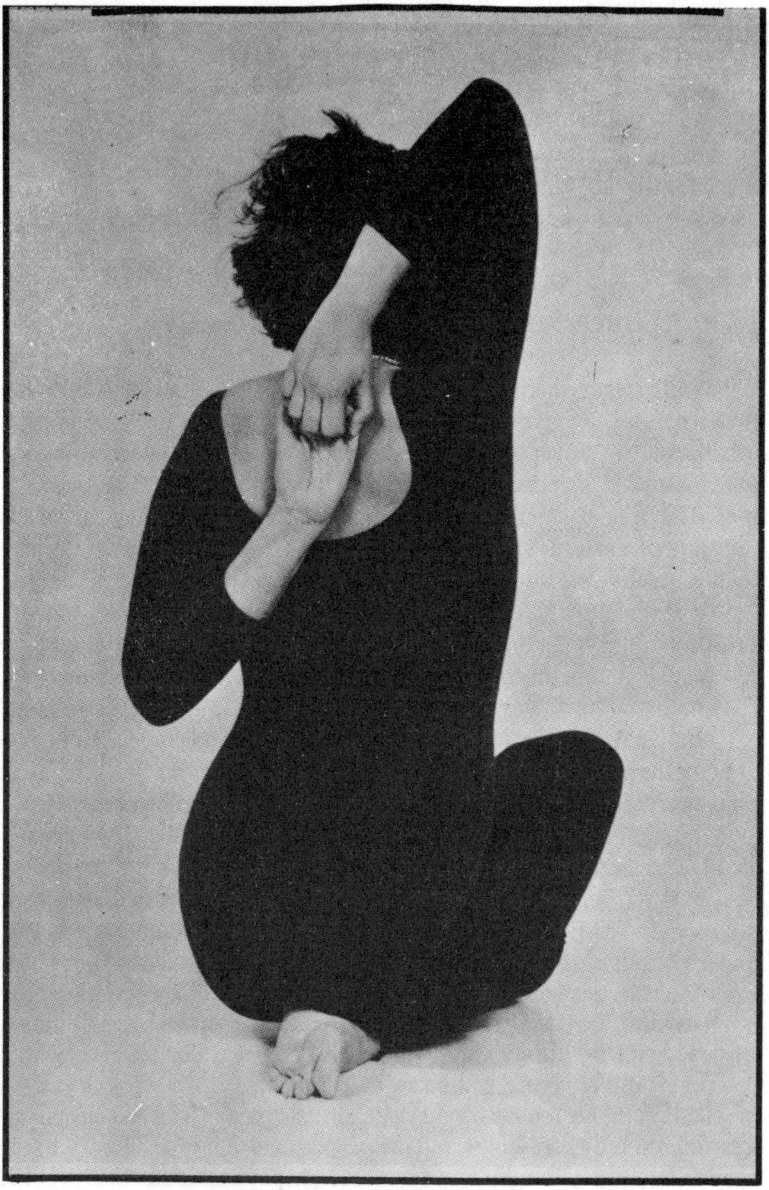

3

UNDERSTANDING OF ASANA: CARE OF THE BODY

3.1 BACKGROUND TO ASANAS (Postural Training)

In the early stages, there were very few (only five) meditative postures for the purpose of meditation and concentration which naturally required a static posture in sitting position. In all such postures, the lower extremities were to be so arranged as to form the base of a triangle with the head as the apex. The spine has to be erect and there is no pressure on any part of the body so that it affords utmost facility for free breathing. There are twenty-eight meditative postures now from which one can choose a posture as per one's convenience. In the past, the search for the ultimate truth was the objective of the yogis and for this they wanted to sit in meditation for long durations. But sometimes, they found they were incapable of pursuing this. They realised that there was the problem of disease not being at ease with oneself. People were suffering because of ill-health and they were not able to sit for the practice of meditation long enough. Since this was coming in the way of their progress, certain yogis who were health educationists, took to investigation and inquired into the true nature of disease. They discovered two to three primary causes. They first came across mul, i.e. impurities. It is the retention of impurities resulting in the accumulation of metabolites which create toxic conditions and the body is enervated. This impairs health and creates an obstacle. They studied and came to know that when the body is pure and clean and uncongested and the nervous energy is not lacking, they can sit for long hours for concentration and meditation without distraction. Another thing they observed was that the body would deteriorate if it remained stationary and was not given any activity. Even the smallest tissue, if not used, became virtually dead. This was atrophy of muscles set in by disuse – which means partial death in a cell, in a tissue or in an organ. Shri Yogendraji says, "All the parts maintain their level of efficiency by use and lose their function by disuse – this is a biological fundamental." The yogis found that elasticity and the activity process of the body, its circulatory, respiratory, digestive and eliminative processes have to be maintained in an efficient form to ensure normal healthy functioning of the organism. But the self-renovating processes are set in motion in the living organisms solely by functional charges through stimulation which has to be provided by suitable activity in the form of exercise and training to our neuro-muscular system. In short, asanas which were primarily meant for meditation were supplemented with a large number of other postures called cultural or therapeutic postures. That is how the physical education movement was started by our ancient life-scientists who were Hatha yogis. They found that the human body was to be kept at a perfect level to help in the achievement of higher levels of consciousness and to achieve the ultimate goal of KAIVALYA (absoluteness).

It works through a comprehensive programme for the care of the body, good health and longevity which brings about postural training through therapeutic asanas, hygiene, sanitation, auto-immunisation and dietetics – all contributing to perfect, positive and sedate health. Now, there are eighty-four known and recognised asanas, out of which twenty-eight are meditative postures. It is very difficult to tell how many are original, how many fictitious and how many innovated.

3.2 ANCIENT METHOD

The ancient yogies with their spiritual goal, had enormous internal power and strong will. Living in a forest, leading a carefree life and with plenty of time at their disposal, they could afford to spend even half a day on such practices and on hygienic processes. These postures involved all the rigours and hardships since each asana was performed traditionally with as much as three hours in a static condition. Any such traditional programme of doing asanas would be most uneconomical, inadvisable and beyond the normal course in the modern conditions of life.

3.3 PROPER REORIENTATION AND SELECTION

The Yoga Institute of Santa Cruz by its half a century of research work, laboratory tests and clinical investigations tried to find out what the essential asanas for the modern man are. After proper screening and scientific evaluation, they selected about twenty postures for the care of the skeleton, muscles and physical body, and graded them from simple to moderately hard to suit all age groups. Static-cum-dynamic variations of asanas were evolved which have proved very exhilarating for the modern man and woman when skilfully performed. They are not vigorous or strenuous, they give one the maximum result in minimum time in the most economical manner with least expenditure of energy.

3.4 ASANAS AS A TOTAL BODY PHENOMENON

The development of the organic system is of great importance as it affects the various internal organs, stimulates them and increases their efficiency, securing perfect health. The method of performing asanas are based on rhythmical alternate contraction and relaxation or stretch and relaxation, of a large group of muscles so as to stimulate circulation, develop elasticity of the body and revitalise and rejuvenate all our internal organs so as to yield the maximum in the general well-being of the individual. Two important areas in the trunk are much emphasized and they are the spine and the abdomen. Besides, the methods affect various nerve centres in control of muscles of the trunk to increase the health and efficiency of the nervous system.

3.5 THE BASIC IDEAL

The common man believes in muscle culture. In Yoga the level is much raised and you should try to understand what is aimed at by the discipline of the body through postural training.

The basic idea is that the structural integrity of the complex human organism – functions of various organs and systems –has to be maintained in health as in disease. All leading scientists hold that the great integrating and coordinating system is the nervous system, which covers each and every part of the human organism from the various organs to the tiniest muscle. You know what happens if the nerve going to a given muscle is destroyed – the muscle fails to respond. "The dynamics of the nervous system, correlated by bioenergy, is the specialized knowledge that the yogis have and therefore they were able to gain control over all involuntary functions of the body, even to the point of suspended animation." In all yoga exercises and processes, the main stress is on the growth, development, control and purification of the nervous system (nadi shuddhi) which affect not only the various internal organs purposefully but also tend towards poise and mental health. This is the basic ideal.

3.6 THE METHOD

The method employed has been on the habitual exercise of effort-cum-endurance by means of neuro-muscular training. This acts as a series of coordinated phases with alternate stretching and contraction of the muscles, providing the necessary stimulation which is organically vital and helps to retain the tonicity and elasticity of the muscular system.

3.7 AREAS COVERED

3.7.1 Spine

Primary importance is given to the merudanda or the spinal column. It is not merely the main support of the body and head but also encases the spinal cord, the most vital part of the central nervous system which passes through the spinal column. A defective spinal column obviously interferes with the nervous system and the health and mental activity are adversely affected. Any course of physical training designed to exercise the spine should necessarily take into account –

(i) the normal adjustments of the spinal vertebrae;
(ii) increased spinal circulation;
(iii) the tonicity of the trunk muscles to hold the spine in its proper position;
(iv) the relief from muscular and nervous strain; and
(v) correcting faulty postures.

The spinal column is especially attended by vertical, lateral, posterior, anterior and torsional stretches, basically to strengthen the various muscles supporting the spine and to keep up its flexibility and suppleness.

3.7.2 Abdomen

The abdominal cavity contains various internal organs like the stomach, liver, spleen, pancreas, intestines, etc. Effort is directed through increased intra-abdominal pressure to ensure their proper functioning. It helps in peristaltic movement, relieves constipation, a sluggish liver, gases, and improves the assimilative and eliminative processes. Besides, these abdominal exercises keep up the tonicity of the abdominal muscles and reduce obesity.

3.7.3 Extremities

It exercises various joints of locomotion to keep up their mobility and to some extent exercises arms and legs.

3.7.4 Exercises to Special Parts

Exercises to neck and head, thereby affecting the important organ, the brain. Certain head-low postures have the wholesome effect of gravity pressure on the various organs of the body above the waist including the vital endocrine glands.

Scientific Classification of ASANAS as evolved at the Yoga Institute:

84 ASANAS

28 MEDITATIVE   56 CULTURAL OR THERAPEUTIC ASANAS

SPINE   ABDOMEN   EXTREMITIES   HEAD-LOW

3.8 A FEW IMPORTANT FEATURES

A slow static-cum-dynamic variation has been evolved where the breathing rhythm (Yogendra rhythm) is ideally coordinated with physical movement, giving you greater hygienic benefit, harmony and ease in performance besides eliminating any chance of respiratory maladjustment.

These are basically exercises of endurance to build up your stamina and resisting power. The neuro-muscular training, affecting the internal organs through the process of functional changes, brings desirable physiological changes contributing to the organismic activity; in other words, maintaining homeostasis like a balance.

3.9 EFFECT ON VARIOUS SYSTEMS

All these factors would result in affecting the various systems which are interrelated and coordinated by the Nervous System.

3.9.1 Muscular System

1. Helps to retain the tonicity and elasticity of the Muscular System.
2. Develops harmonious postures, making the body supple and agile in its movements.
3. Maintains natural balance and coordination between the various parts of the body as well as the internal organs.

3.9.2 Respiratory System

1. Special Yogendra breathing rhythm to be followed scientifically in the performance of asanas skilfully. Manipulation of nervous energy (Prana) through important nerve centres which has its healing power.
2. Helps to increase the supply of oxygen.
3. Increases the breathing capacity.
4. Respiratory harmony is maintained

3.9.3 Circulatory System

1. Increases the circulation of blood throughout the body.
2. The oxygen-carrying capacity of the blood is augmented.

3.9.4 Digestive System

1. Improves assimilative and eliminative processes.
2. Helps in two common ailments of indigestion and constipation.

ASANA (postural training programme) has a TOTAL BODY PHENOMENON where kinesiological, physiological and psychological factors are taken into account not only to re-establish HOMEOSTASIS but also to help in mental, moral and psychic development. We must not forget that in yoga, the physical body merely serves as the instrument of education for the mind.

3.10 YOGA AND NON-YOGA TYPES OF PHYSICAL CULTURE

There is a vital difference between the two according to Shri Yogendraji.

YOGA	NON-YOGA
1. Static Comparatively static-cum-dynamic based on the principle of relaxation	**Repetitive** Movement repetitive based on tension.
2. Organismic Development of organic system with increased efficiency of the assimilation and eliminative process. Especially tones up vital organs.	**Muscular** Movement directed more to skeletal muscles.
3. Anabolic Uses energy to a minimum without causing fatigue or oxygen debt.	**Katabolic** Involves more expenditure of energy.
4. Sedative Has a soothing effect on the nervous system.	**Organistic** Contributes to nervous agitation.
5. Subjective Leads to inwardness and self-control.	**Objective** Leads to extrovertness, exhibitionism and encourages competitive spirit.
6. Extra-Mundane Contributes to mental purity and makes a person extra-mundane.	**Mundane** Not conducive to mental hygiene – actually decentralizes the mind and makes a person mundane.

3.11 THE SIMPLE SCHEME

The scheme of 'Yoga Better Living Courses' in the book is divided into two parts – the first 12 BL basic course common for both men and women and the second 24 BL general course for men and separately a special course for women which includes practices especially beneficial for them. Sita Devi Yogendra says, "The cyclic changes and increased organic responsibilities of motherhood require specific physical preparation commensurate with her needs." There are different postures for men and women because there are anatomical and psychological differences which, in a scientific study, cannot be ignored.

The selection of the asanas even in the first 12 BL Course (Basic) has been carefully made so that each part of the body receives proper care and sufficient exercise in a short period of 30 to 40 minutes. Of course, the second 24 BL Course (General) covers many more practices and will take 40 to 60 minutes. Combination of postures, however, are graded from simple to moderately hard. Special emphasis is given to the spine and abdomen. Every one must first take the basic course of 12 practices. It is simple, safe and can easily be taken up even by those who have minor health problem, weak constitution or suffering from STRESS CONDITION. Practise this course for two months as per Guide Table and once the body has developed certain flexibility and the abdomen muscles have toned up a bit, then alone pick up, intelligently, practices that are covered in the general course of 24 practices.

How to commence the 12 BL Course, the weekly time table is given for each day of the week. In the second week, you follow the proper sequence mentioned in the guide table.

3.12 PROGRAMME OF LEARNING: Ist Week

3.12.1 Ist Week

Ist DAY:

1. Sukhasana
2. Talasana II, III variation
3. Konasana I variation
4. Vajrasana

2nd DAY:

5. Yogendra Pranayama 4 (Y.P. No. 4)
6. Wakrasana

3rd DAY:

7. Bhujangasana
8. Tratak a & b

4th DAY:

9. Yogendra Pranayama 1 (Y.P. No. 1)
10. Yoga Mudra

5th DAY:

11. Talasana I variation
12. Konasana II variation
13. Yogendra Nishpanda Bhava

6th DAY:

14. Do Jalaneti followed by all the practices so far learnt.

7th DAY:

15. To add Savasana (complete relaxation) after the performance of all the above practices.

3.12.2 2nd Week: Follow this sequence broadly:

1. MEDITATIVE POSTURES – Sukhasana/Vajrasana alter nate day.
2. CULTURAL ASANAS
   a) The standing postures
   b) The sitting postures
   c) The lying-down postures
3. BREATHING PROCESS
   A) Abdominal breathing (Y.P. No. 4)
   b) Yogendra Pranayama 1 (Y.P. No. 1)
4. PSYCHOSOMATIC PRACTICES FOR RELAXATION
   a) Yogendra Nishpanda Bhava Alternate Day OR
   b) Savasana

3.13 GUIDELINES TO PERFORMANCE

Most of the asanas are performed with short pause and slow rhythm and this is termed as static-cum-dynamic variation of asanas. For the first two weeks give very little pause of retention or suspension. Treat them as a slow series of rhythmic movements accompanied by either inhalation or exhalation – a well coordinated exercise as prescribed in a dynamic way. In the third week get to the habit of giving a static respiratory pause of 4 seconds of retention or suspension. Gradually increase this pause period from 4 to a maximum of 6 seconds in two months time to derive maximum benefit as mentioned in the Guide Table.

In this manner we coordinate and maintain the correct breathing rhythm with the performance of each asana. The movements have to be slow, free from vigorous effort and strain and avoid unnecessary pulls of muscles, so that the antagonistic muscles are relaxed at the proper time and thus do not impede the functioning of the acting muscles. It reduces tension and fatigue. Each asana is attitude-bound and requires conscious association of the mind with the varying movements of the body, performed with maximum precision and will-power. All this is intended to achieve proper coordination, balance and control.

Remember the components of Yogendra Rhythm, a process of breathing, are:

INH : INHALATION	(puraka)
RET : RETENTION	(kumbhaka)
EXH : EXHALATION	(recaka)
SUS : SUSPENSION	(sunyaka)

and they have been worked out systematically on the basis of 1:2:1 i.e., one matra (count) of inhalation is followed by two matra (counts) of retention/ suspension and inhalation and exhalation are equal. This has been laid down by Shri Gorakhnath, one of the greatest exponents of Yoga.

3.14 GUIDELINES TO PERFORMANCE

1. One should wear loose garments while doing the exercises.
2. It is good to attend to the call of nature before starting yogic practices.
3. Yogic practice can be done before or after a bath in the morning or in the evening before dinner or 3 hrs after meals.
4. A cup of milk/tea/fruit juice can be taken if so desired twenty minutes before the practices.
5. For ladies postural exercises which involve intra-abdominal compression should be discontinued for the first three days of menstruation and also during advanced pregnancy.
6. Routine practice to be performed always after conditioning the

mind in one of the meditative postures for at least 5 minutes followed by cultural asanas in standing, sitting and lying-down position etc. In the end do one of the relaxation practices.

7. It is important to select yogic postures from 24 BL course to suit your capacity (Refer Guide Table), needs and the time at your disposal but a minimum of 30 to 40 minutes should be devoted to yoga routine practice. Practise 12 BL course for two months before you pick up practices from 24 BL course (Appendix 2).
8. Select first a simple one from each of the practicals under Section 2.2 and 3.7, given in the book and slowly add up as you progress in the 24 BL course (Appendix 2).
9. Remember, however good a posture may be, you should not overdo it or strain yourself. There should be no muscular strain or unbearable pressure upon the internal organs.
10. Do practice of Y. Pranayama No. 1 or Yogic complete breathing every morning and evening.
11. It is advisable to do Yogendra Nishpanda Bhava after lunch in your office for 10/15 minutes, sitting in an easy chair. It will keep your mind alert and sharp for the rest of the day.
12. After the whole day's work when you reach home, do abdominal breathing in lying down position (Y. Pranayama No. 4) followed by Savasana for ten minutes.
13. At night before going to bed do the practice of Bhavana (reflection) as mentioned in Section 13.5 and then do partial Savasana for sound sleep.
14. Do your routine practice regularly and with proper mental attitude.

4

EXERCISES FOR THE SPINE

4.1 VERTICAL STRETCHING

4.1.1 Talasana (*The Palmae Pose*) and its three variations

(i) POSTURE: Standing erect with feet apart, raise arm or both the arms over your head and also heels simultaneously with inhalation.

(ii) METHOD: (a) First variation

1. Stand erect, feet parallel, about 9" distance between the feet, and spine straight.
2. Raise one arm from the front and both the heels simultaneously, inhaling, arm taut, touching the ear with palm inwards.
3. Reach maximum stretch position, maintain for some seconds in retention (Fig. 5a).
4. Rotate the arm backwards and downwards, slowly exhaling, and heels to come down simultaneously. Repeat with the other arm.
5. Do it four times with alternate use of arm.

   (b) Second variation (Fig. 5b).

6. Do exactly as above, with both the arms.

   (c) Third variation (Fig. 5c).

7. Raise both the arms from the sides and join the two palms over the head.

(iii) RHYTHM:

INH	RET	EXH	SUS
3 :	6 :	3 :	3

(iv) FREQUENCY: Each variation to be performed four times.

(v) BENEFITS: Stretches the entire body; the rhythmic breathing helps expansion of lungs and develops respiratory muscles; exercises and massages the abdominal viscera indirectly; increases height (up to a certain age); vertical stretch of spine. It increases neuro-muscular coordination.

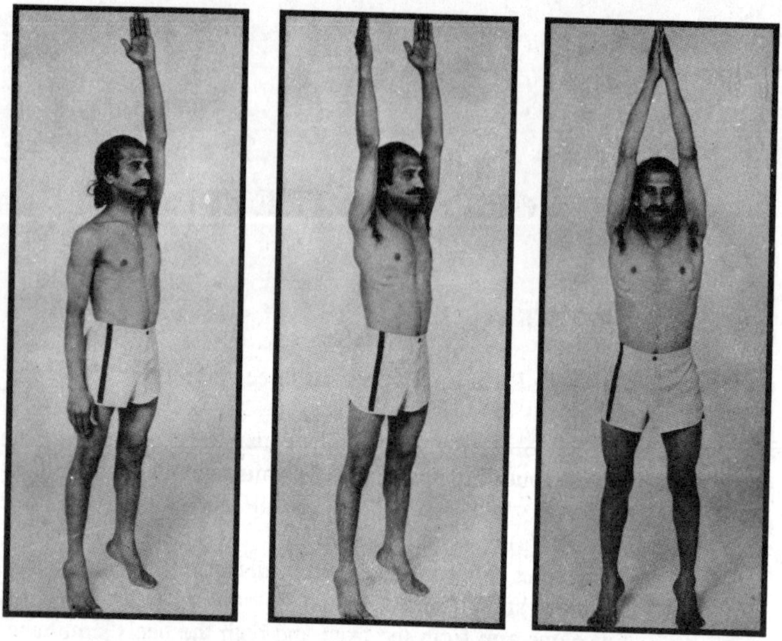

4.1.2 **Yastikasana** (*Stick Pose*) Easy technique of vertical stretch

(i) POSTURE: Lying straight on your back, fully stretch both the arms and the lower extremities in the opposite directions.

(ii) METHOD

1. Lie on your back, take your arms fully extended over the head but touching the floor in an easy and relaxed manner (Fig. 6a).

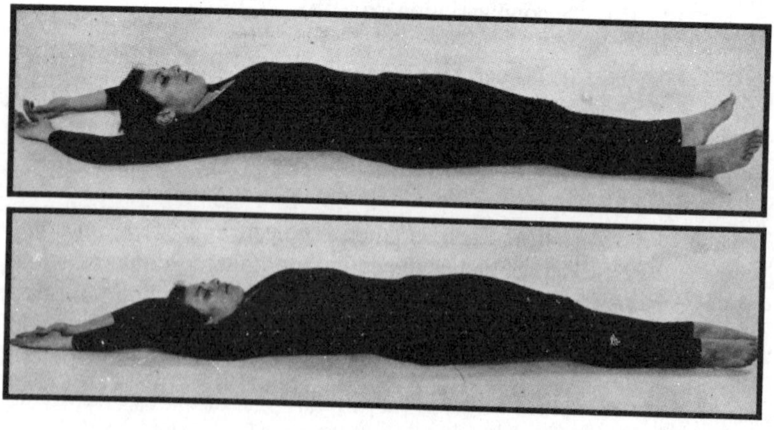

2. Stretch the body fully, slowly, while inhaling - arms and hands and legs and feet pulled in opposite directions as far as possible, with 3 seconds of inhalation (Fig. 6b).
3. Retain this stretch position for 6 seconds.
4. Release the tension and return to non-stretching with exhalation for 3 seconds.

(iii) RHYTHM:

INH	RET	EXH
3 :	6 :	3

(iv) FREQUENCY: Repeat 4 times.

(v) BENEFITS: Maximum stretching of the body without undue straining; increases height (up to a certain age); corrects the normal interspacing of the vertebrae; good for backache.

4.1.3 Parvatasana (*Mountain Pose*) and its variations

(i) POSTURE: Sitting in a meditative pose of Padmasana or, if that is not possible, in Sukhasana, raise the hands and arms upward, above the head and stretch fully with inhalation. Do movements of bending on all four sides.

(ii) METHOD (a) *First variation*

1. Sit in Sukhasana/Padmasana and raise your hands and

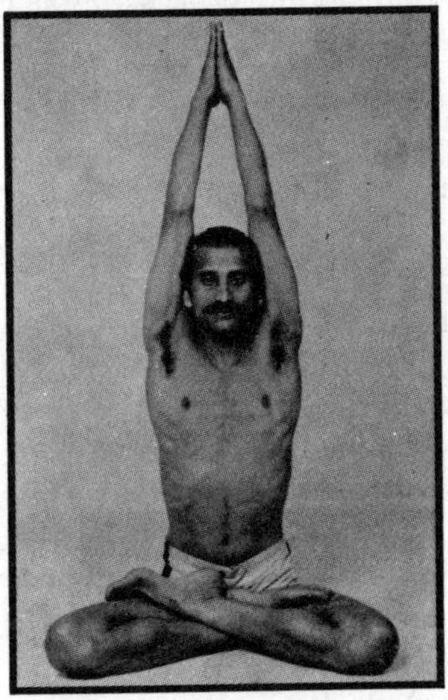

arms while inhaling with palms joined and pressed against each other or interlace the fingers (Fig. 7a).

2. Give a full upward vertical stretch (Fig. 7b).
3. Maintain pause for 6 seconds in retention.

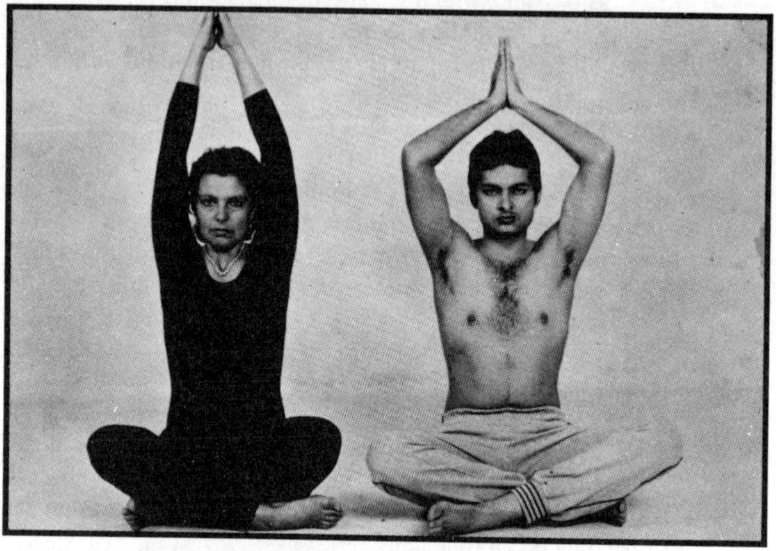

4. Return to starting position with exhalation.
5. While performing this asana, keep your eyes fixed on any object in front of you.

(iii) RHYTHM: INH RET EXH

3 : 6 : 3

(iv) FREQUENCY : Repeat three times.

(b) *Second Variation*

1. After giving upward stretch to hands and arms, in the pause period of retention.

(i) Sway forward and lean backward and come to the starting

(c) *Third Variation*

1. In the pause period of retention as above,

(ii) bend sideward to the right and then bend sideward to the left (Fig. 7c).

Note: Do these movements (i) & (ii) on the four sides separately and alternately.

(v) RHYTHM: INH RET EXH

3 : 6 : 3

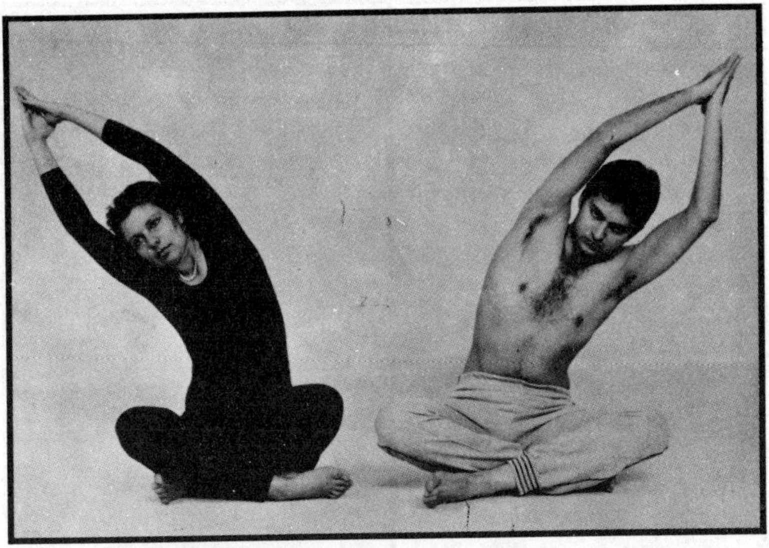

(vi) FREQUENCY: Repeat three times (i) & (ii)

(vii) BENEFITS

I variation: Corrects minor postural defects of the spine; helps reduce flabbiness of the abdominal walls; exercises the less used muscles of the waist zone.

II & III variations: Stretches all sets of muscles supporting the trunk; helps in ptosis, stasis and prolapse of the uterus; results in indirect massage to internal organs; loosens the hips.

4.2 L ATERAL STRETCHING

4.2.1 Konasana (*Angle Pose*)

(i) POSTURE: With feet apart, bending sideward from waist alternately with inhalation.

(ii) METHOD: Correct standing position; feet parallel, 20" to 24" apart.

First variation

1. Place one hand on waist and the other on the side of the thigh (Fig. 8a).
2. Turn head (profile). Bend sideward, inhaling, slide the hand on side downward and hand on waist upward towards the armpit (Fig. 8b). No bending of body forward or backward and no bending of knees.

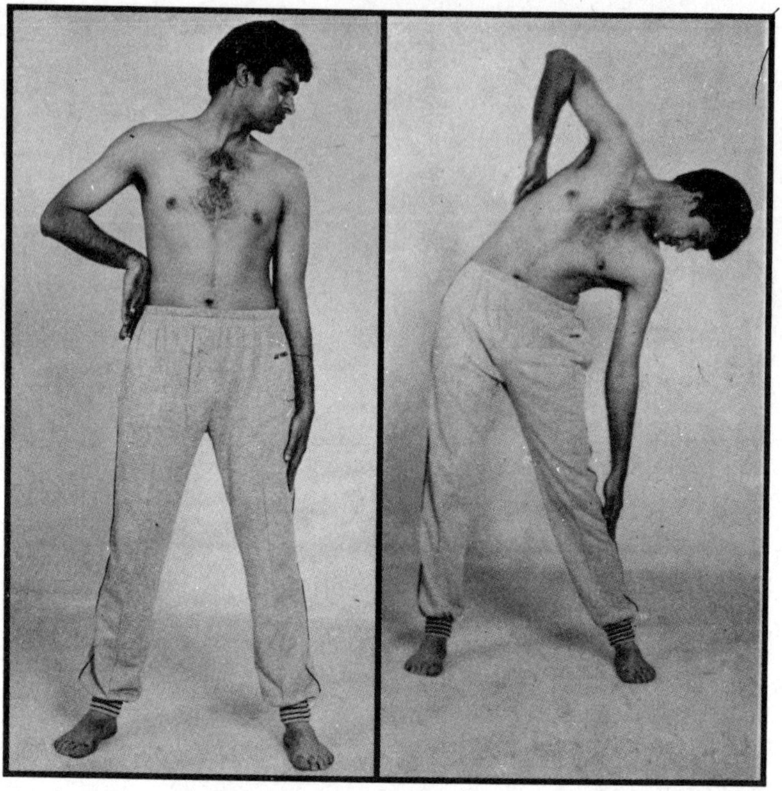

3. Reach your fingers to knee and towards ankle.
4. Check simultaneous sliding of both hands - position of head and body.
5. Return to normal exhaling.
6. Turn your head to the other side and repeat.

Second variation

1. Raise one arm taut, touching ear, the other arm on the side of thigh (Fig. 9a).
2. Reach your fingers to knee or towards ankle - no bending of body forward or backward and no bending of knees (Fig. 9b).
3. Return to normal exhaling.
4. Repeat on the other side.

(iii) RHYTHM: INH RET EXH

3 : 6 : 3

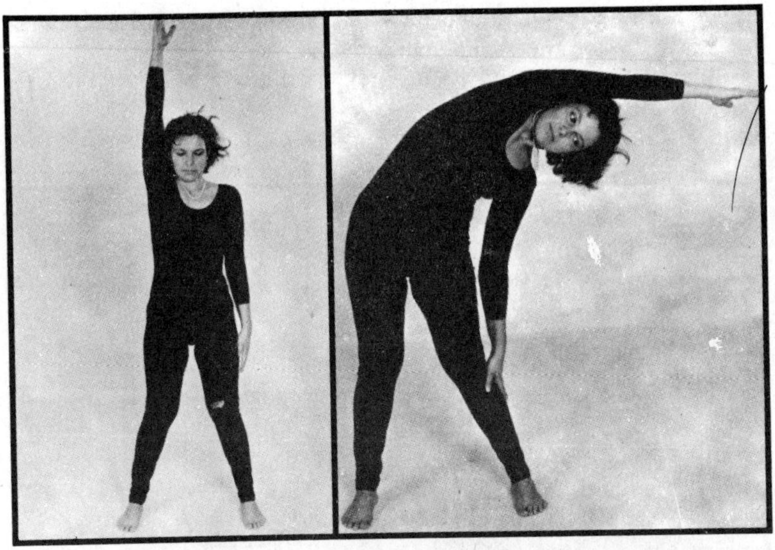

(iv) FREQUENCY: Three times alternately bending on each side.

(v) BENEFITS: Lateral stretching of spine; exercises the less-used muscles of the sides and waist; compresses and massages the body organs like liver, stomach, kidneys large intestine etc.; prevents backache; removes fat and obesity.

4.3 POSTERIOR STRETCHING (Forward Bending Postures)

4.3.1 Yoga Mudra (*The Symbol of Yoga*) in Sukhasana

(i) POSTURE: Sitting in Sukhasana, hold the wrist of one hand with the other at the back and bending forward to touch knees alternately and then bending forward in the centre.

(ii) METHOD

1. Sit in Sukhasana. Hold wrist of right hand by left hand - inhale.
2. Check spine and neck which should be straight.
3. Bend to touch the right knee by the tip of your nose, with exhalation (Fig. 10).
4. Check the back - do not strain to touch.
5. Return to starting position with inhalation.
6. Repeat on left knee.

7. Repeat, bending forward to touch the floor in front between the knees with your forehead.

(iii) RHYTHM: EXH SUS INH

	EXH	SUS	INH
	3:	6:	3

(iv) FREQUENCY: Four rounds

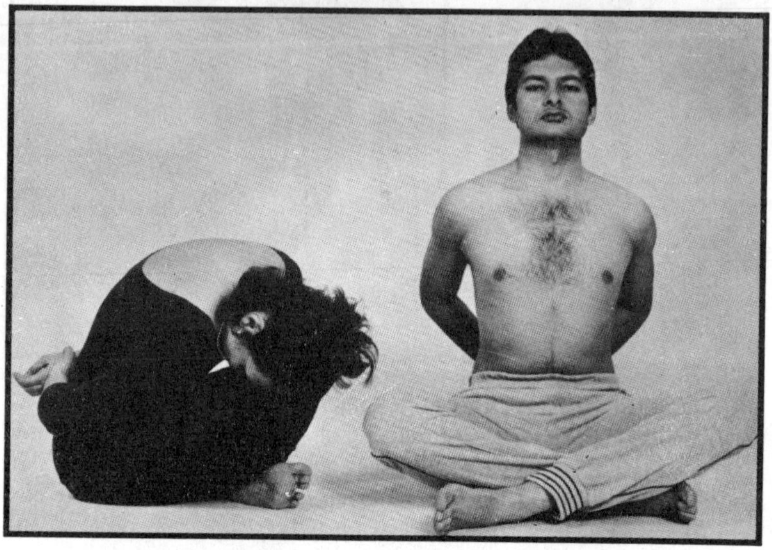

(v) BENEFITS: Posterior stretching of the spine; lateral stretching of almost all the posterior muscles of the trunk and neck; intra-abdominal compression gives a gentle massage to the internal organs; improves circulation of blood in the face and head region; improves elimination of toxic wastes; leads to a relaxed passive state of consciousness.

4.3.2 Trikonasana (*Triangle Pose*)

(i) POSTURE: Stand upright with feet together, raise your hands and bend forward from the waist, with exhalation.

(ii) METHOD

1. Stand erect, feet together, raise your hands over your head, inhaling.
2. While exhaling, bend forward the body above waist.
3. Try to touch the toes with fingers, no bending of knees, spine and neck kept horizontal (Fig. 11).

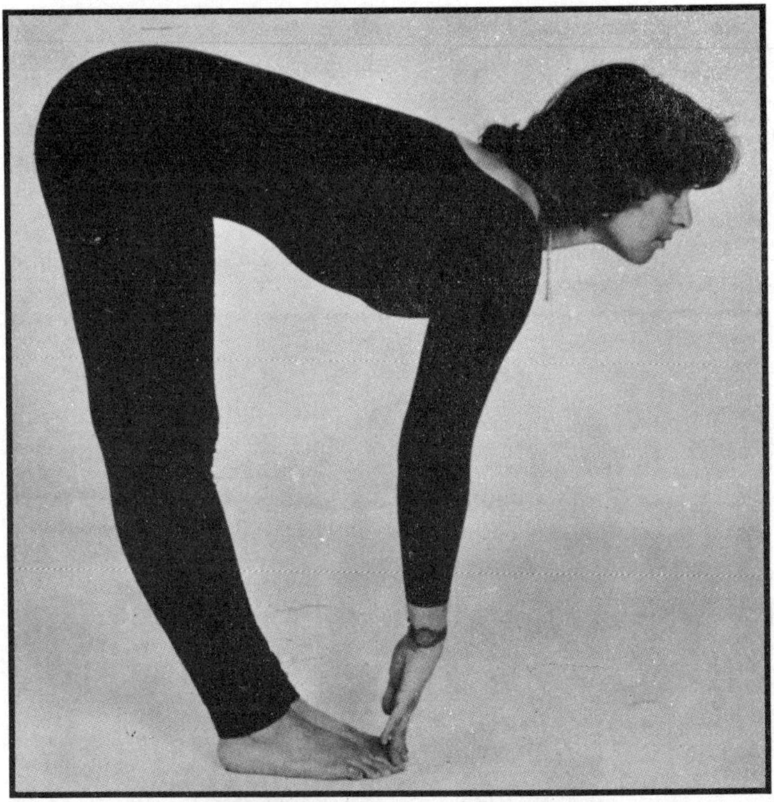

4. Fix your gaze on the tip of the nose.
5. Return to original position inhaling.

(iii) RHYTHM: EXH SUS INH
3 : 6 : 3

(iv) FREQUENCY: Repeat five times without pause.

(v) BENEFITS: Posterior stretching of the spine; increase in flexibility of the waist; exercises the hips; stretching of the muscles of legs and arms; hamstring muscles are strengthened; good effect on the sciatic nerve; corrects faulty posture-habits by intra-abdominal compression.

(vi) FOR THE BEGINNERS: Keep 3" distance between feet, bend forward slowly from the waist, keeping head downwards. Give gentle downward pressure but don't bend the knees. As flexibility improves, the fingers may touch the ground or you may even be able to place the palms flat on the floor.

4.3.3 Hastapadasana (*Arm-leg Pose*)

(i) METHOD

1. Same as Trikonasana but in this case while bending forward with exhalation, try to catch hold of the ankles with hands, keeping the head downward, gradually draw the head nearer the knees (Fig. 12).
2. Maintain the pose for four seconds in suspension and return to original position, inhaling.

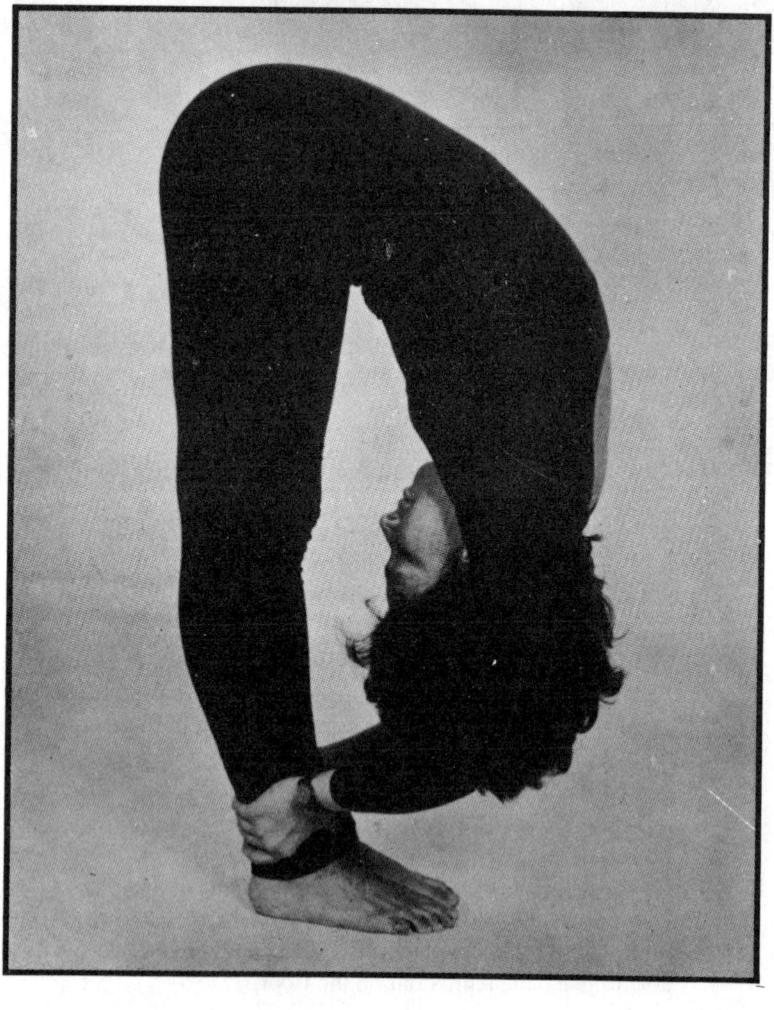

(ii) RHYTHM: EXH SUS INH
3 : 6 : 3

(iii) FREQUENCY: Five times.

Note: Women should discontinue this for the first three days of menstruation and also during advanced pregnancy. those having high blood pressure or heart trouble (men as well as women) should not do Hastapadasana or Trikonasana.

(iv) FOR THE BEGINNERS: Avoid haste and jerks. As the suppleness of your spine permits, try to touch first the toes or the floor after bending forward - try every day till you are able to reach the ankles with your hands. In the final position, hold the ankles tightly with the respective hands, fold the arms near the elbows and try to draw the head nearer the knees (See Fig. 15). Return slowly to the starting position while inhaling. Beginners should practise it daily for a few weeks in the evening but should not overdo it. It is essential, when bending forward, to reach the toes, floor or ankles, to keep the feet together and the knees straight and not to bend the legs at all, otherwise its beneficial effects are lost.

(v) BENEFITS: Same as those from Trikonasana. Results in intra-abdominal pressure; extreme stretching of the posterior muscles; good effect on the abdomen, waistline and the hips and helps in reducing unhealthy fat.

4.3.4 Janusirasana (*The Head-Knee Pose*)

(i) POSTURE: With one leg stretched, bend the other leg in a manner that the sole of the foot touches the opposite thigh. Bend down your trunk and head towards the knee with exhalation.

(ii) METHOD

1. In a sitting position, stretch out the left leg and bend the right leg in a manner that the sole touches the left thigh, with the heel exerting pressure on the perineum (Fig. 13a).
2. Keep the trunk and head erect and breathe in.
   FOR THE BEGINNERS
3. With exhalation, bend the head forward and downward towards the knees and extend forward the forearms and fingers towards the extended left leg as much as is convenient.

4. With inhalation, get back to the starting upright sitting position and straighten the folded leg.
5. Repeat the movements with right leg stretched out.

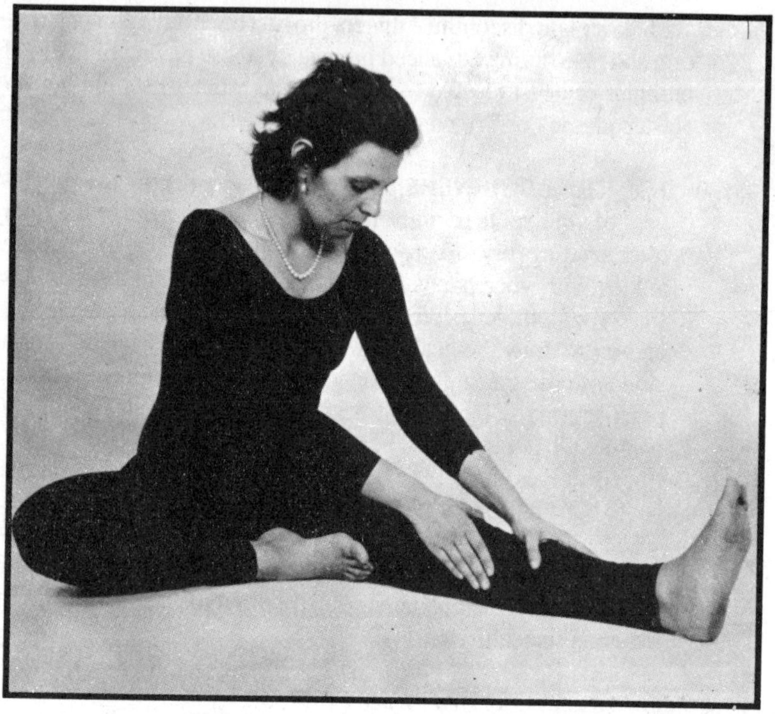

(iii) INSTRUCTION: As the flexibility develops in the process of doing it, lower the elbow, bend down to touch the knee with your forehead, at the same time hold the big toes with your fingers - if this is also possible, then clasp the ball of the left foot with your hands which will stretch your back fully. Remember, the knee must not be lifted from the floor as you bend forward (Fig. 13b).

(iv) RHYTHM: EXH SUS INH
3 : 6 : 3

(v) FREQUENCY: Repeat four times with alternate leg.

(vi) BENEFITS: Good effect on the sciatic nerve and loosens hip joints; stretches the hamstring muscles; improves blood circulation to the head and face; provides relief in intestinal colic and gas

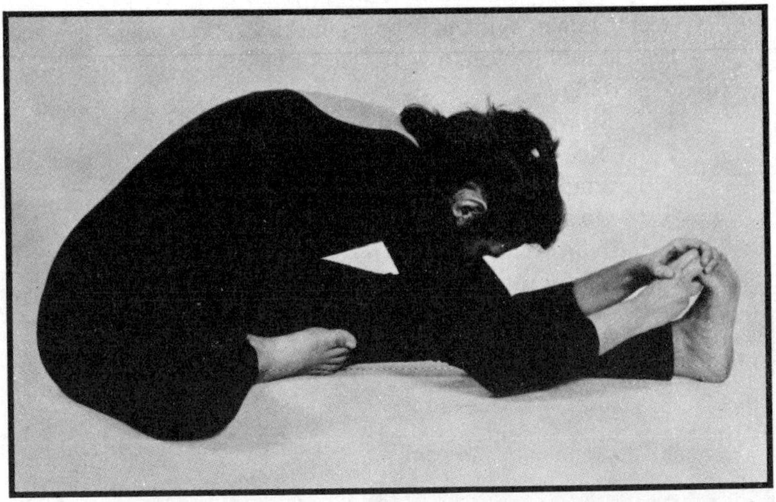

troubles; removes congestion of the liver, spleen and helps the peristalsis of the intestines; prepares for Paschimottanasana.

4.3.5 Paschimottanasana (*The Posterior Stretching Pose*) - the dynamic way*

(i) POSTURE: In sitting position, stretch out your legs in front, with

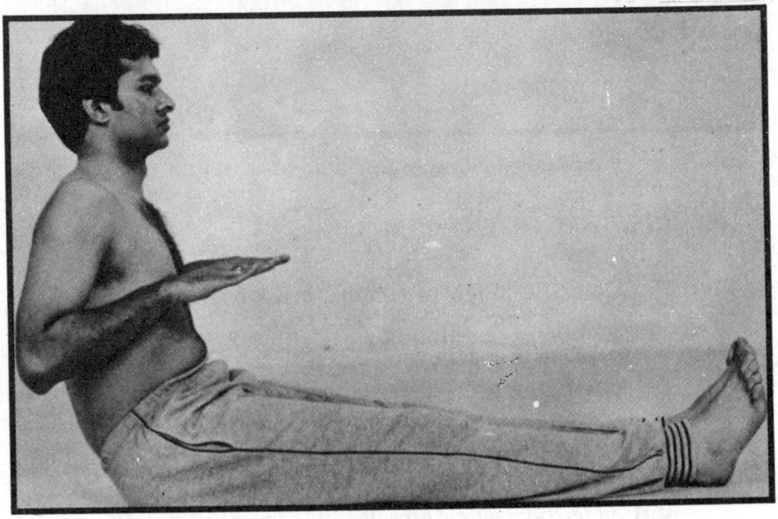

* Static means when the posture is completed, you remain in that position.

feet together. Without bending the knees, bend your trunk and head slowly forward towards the knees while breathing out.

(ii) METHOD

1. Sit with legs stretched, toes turned inwards.
2. Keep both the arms along the sides of the trunk near the armpit.
3. Go slightly back and inhale (Fig. 14a).
4. With exhalation, bend body forward, arms stretched - reach out for toes, bending head down (Fig. 14b).

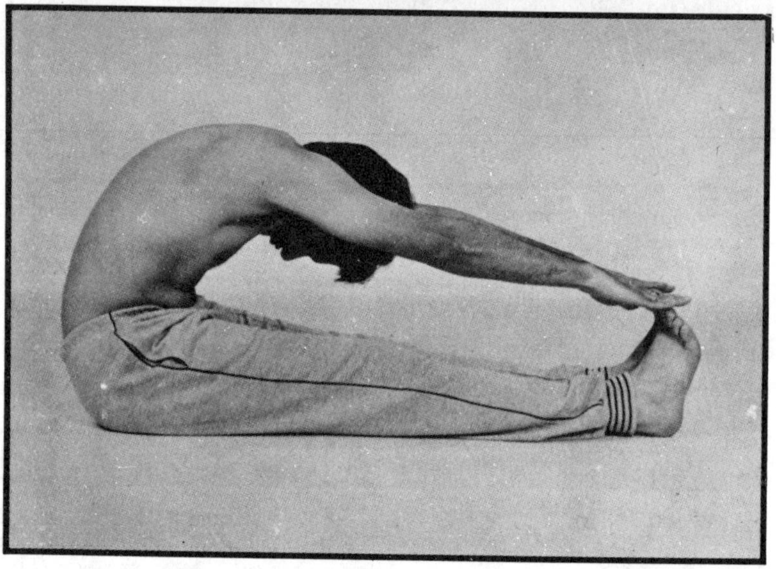

5. Withdraw the arms, inhaling, and return to the original starting position.

(iii) RHYTHM: EXH INH
3 : 3

(iv) FREQUENCY: Eight to ten times in a dynamic way like rowing.

Note: When full palm goes beyond toes with practice hold the toes with the respective fingers and the thumb of either hand. Give pause of suspension of four seconds. Do it only six times.

(vi) BENEFITS: Maximum posterior stretch of the spine; good for stiff spine; tones spinal muscles and nerves and improves considerably; deep intra-abdominal compression; improves digestive

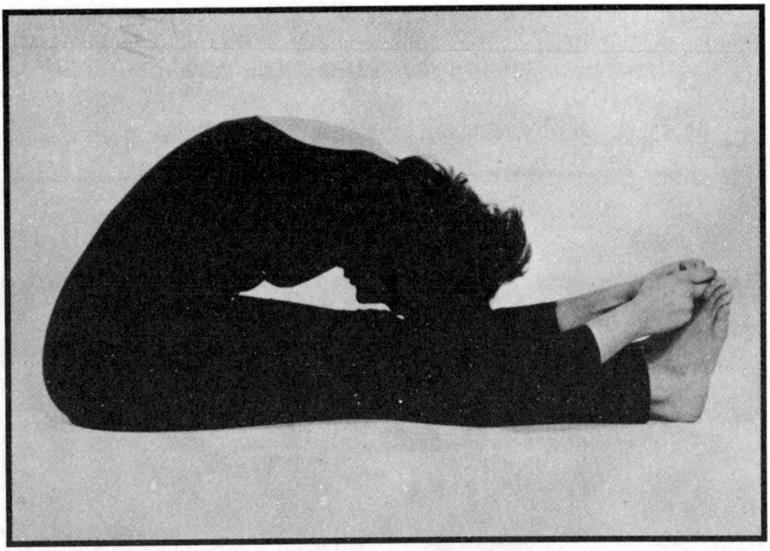

power and relieves constipation; good for those having a low blood pressure; helps to reduce abdominal obesity and fat from hips, buttocks and thighs.

Note: Perform the movement rhythmically and practise slowly in a relaxed manner. With regular practice in a dynamic way, the muscles of the thighs, the hamstring muscles (at the back of the knees) and the back muscles will improve, joints loosen up and the spine becomes more supple. It is a counterpose to Bhujangasana where the spine is stretched in the opposite direction.

(vi) CONTRA-INDICATED: Those who have hernia problem or high blood pressure should avoid it.
People who have undergone any abdominal operation must do it only on doctor's advice.
Women to do its dynamic variation and not in a static position of holding the toes and giving a pause of suspension. Also avoid during menstruation and pregnancy.

4.3.6 Halasana (*The Plough Pose*)

(i) POSTURE: Lie on your back and raise both the legs with inhalation, the buttocks and the lower back held together with the help of both the hands. Take the legs slowly behind your head breathing out so that your toes touch the ground.

(ii) METHOD

1. Lie on your back (supine), arms resting on respective sides.

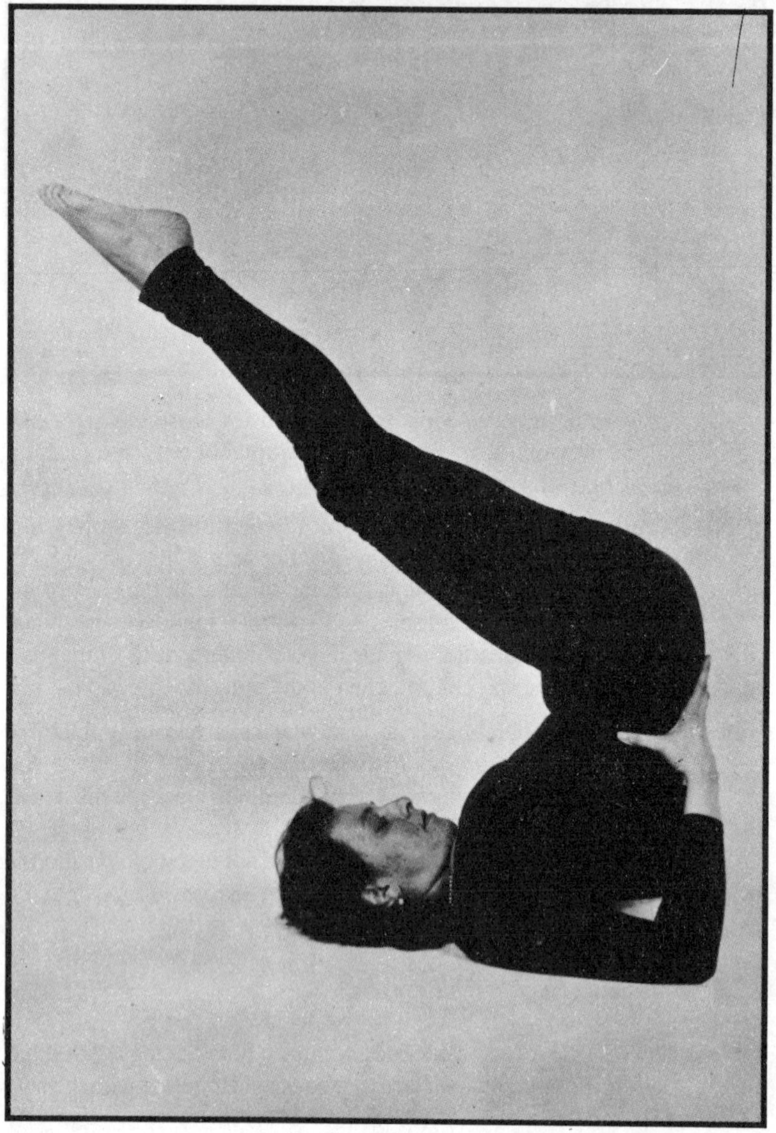

2. Raise both legs slowly without bending the knees, with inhalation.
3. Raise the hips and lower the legs towards the head and then beyond it with slow exhalation (Fig. 15a).
4. Let the toes touch the ground, toes to be kept pointed outward (Fig. 15b) (even if unable to make the feet touch the ground, take them as far as you can without bending the knees).

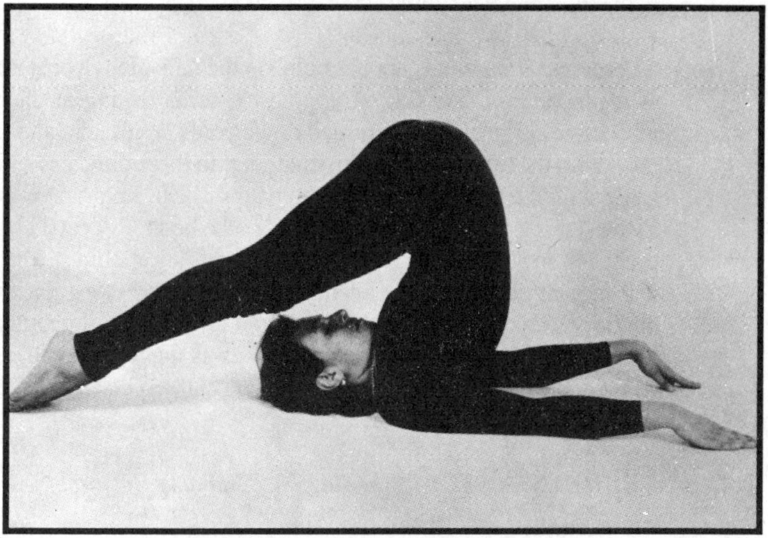

5. Arms to be kept in their original position.
6. Return to starting position with inhalation.

(iii) RHYTHM: INH EXH SUS INH
3 : 3 : 6 : 3

(iv) FREQUENCY: Five rounds.

Note: If it is done in a static manner,* do it only once and in the final static pose, adopt normal slow rhythmic breathing, for not more than two minutes.

(v) BENEFITS: Gives posterior stretch of the spine; healthy effects on the nervous system, digestive systems and the genital organs; effective in eliminating toxemia; good for relieving constipation;

* Static means when the posture is completed, you remain in that position.

corrects sexual debility; corrects menstrual disorders; reduces spinal rigidity; improves the functioning of the thoracic and abdominal viscera and also the blood circulation of the brain; strengthens the supporting muscles and ligaments of the uterus and the ovaries.

(vi) CONTRA-INDICATED: During the first three days of menses and the last five months of pregnancy. Those suffering from prolapse of the uterus or hernia should try it very cautiously (only in the dynamic way with folded or bent legs).

Note: If complete Halasana is not possible, do the half-plough posture as a preparation. Lie flat on your back, arms resting at their respective sides and palms turned downwards. With inhalation, raise both the legs together, perpendicular to the ground or right angle with the body by pressing the palms down. Return slowly to the starting position - exhaling. Relax the body. Repeat 3 to 4 times. As an alternative, one can do it with one leg at a time taking it as high as possible while inhaling keeping the other leg flat on the floor. Repeat with the other leg. Do it three times alternating the legs and then do it with both the legs as mentioned above. Raise and lower the legs as slowly as you can, especially as the legs come close to the floor.

4.4 ANTERIOR STRETCHING (*Backward Bending Postures*)

4.4.1 Bhujangasana (*Snake Pose*)

(i) POSTURE: Lie flat with legs fully stretched out. Raise the upper portion of the body breathing in.

(ii) METHOD

1. Lie on your abdomen, legs stretched, toes pointing outwards and bring the hands just below shoulders (Fig. 16a).

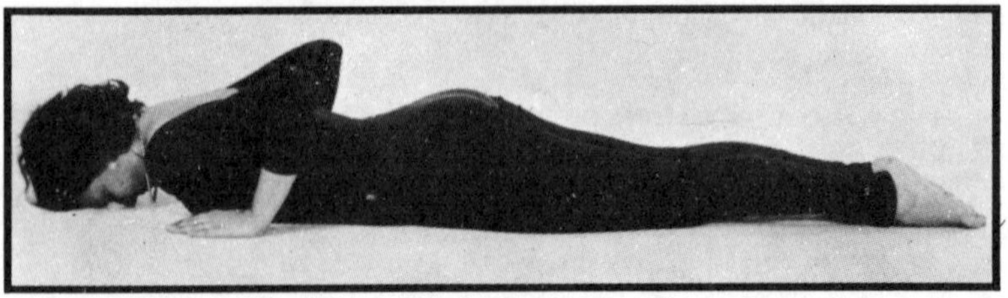

2. With the aid of arms, slowly raise the upper portion of the body above the waist while inhaling (Fig. 16b).

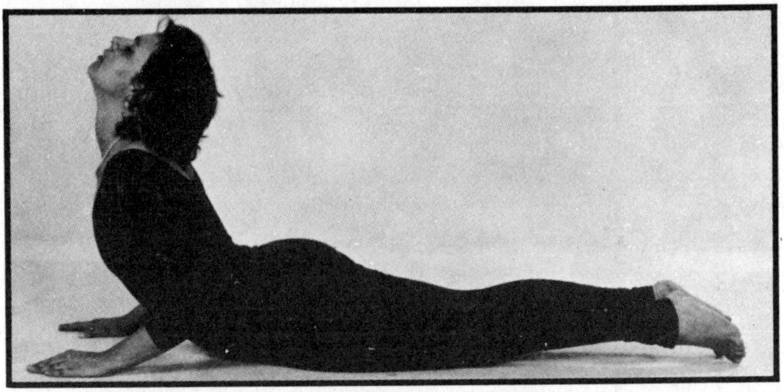

3. Return to starting position - exhaling and rest.

(iii) RHYTHM:

INH		RET		EXH
3	:	6	:	3

(iv) FREQUENCY: Five times.

(v) BENEFITS: Adjusts minor displacements of the vertebrae; exercises and tones the deep muscles supporting the spinal column and the trunk; promotes spinal circulation; provides relief from flatulence and abdominal adhesions.

(vi) CONTRA-INDICATED: During menstruation and advance pregnancy; for hernia and colitis.

4.4.2 **Chakrasana** (*The Wheel Pose*)

(i) POSTURE: Stand with feet apart, raise arms upward. First lean backward with inhalation and then bend forward from the waist with exhalation.

(ii) METHOD

1. Stand with feet apart at 18" to 20". Raise arms upward, interlace the fingers, arms touching the ears (Fig. 17a).
2. Lean backward with inhalation, retain the position for six seconds (Fig. 17b).
3. Bend forward during exhalation with upstretched arms in position - bend head down, do not bend the knees (Fig. 17c).

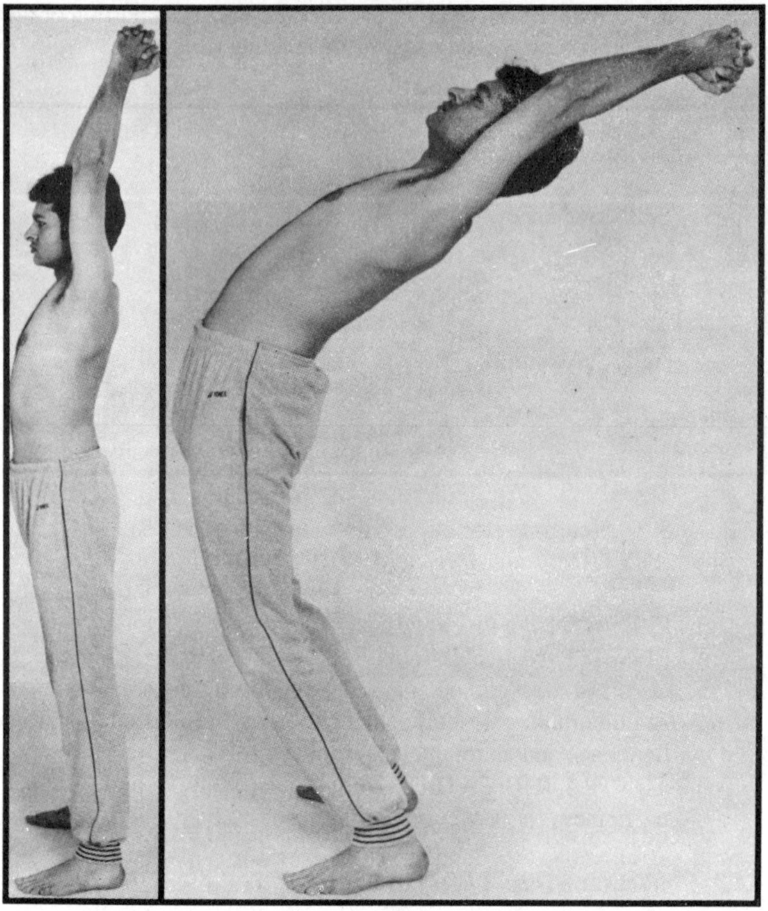

4. Try to touch the ground and later on try to bring the head in contact with the knees.
5. Reverse the whole process during inhalation and come back to the original leaning backward position.

(iii) RHYTHM: INH RET EXH INH
3 : 6 : 3 : 3

(iv) FREQUENCY: Repeat five times.

(v) BENEFITS: Antero-posterior variety; exercises the back muscles and also major and deep abdominal muscles; activates the intestine; exercises the neck and shoulders; good exercise for mid-trunk and spine; activates sluggish liver and improves colon activity.

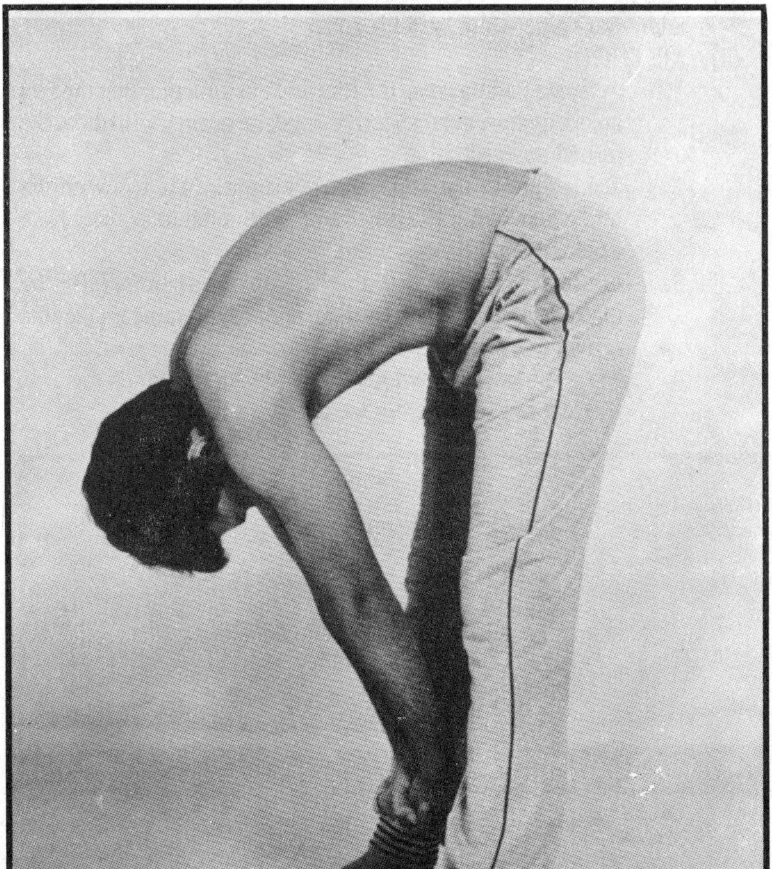

4.4.3 Matsyasana (*The Fish Pose*)

(i) POSTURE: Sitting in Padmasana (the Lotus Pose), lean back and arch your spine while breathing in.

(ii) METHOD

1. Assume Padmasana - the foot-lock in a manner that the feet are set against the respective opposite groins, with the soles turned upward.
2. Taking aid of the arms, throw weight of the trunk on the elbows one after the other and, with inhalation, lean back gradually and lie down flat.
3. Grasp the back of your thighs with your palms, raise the chest and abdomen to form an arch of the spine and let the crown of your head press the floor.
4. Press the knees down gently and bring the hands towards the feet to catch the big toes (Fig. 18).

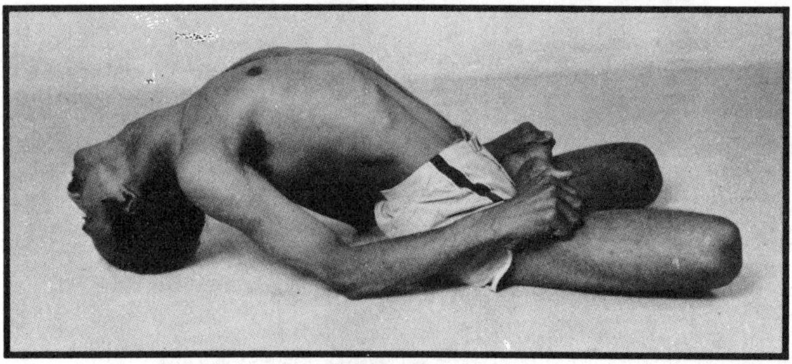

5. Maintain pose retaining the breath for six seconds and return to starting position of Padmasana with exhalation.

(iii) RHYTHM: INH RET EXH
3 : 6 : 3

(iv) FREQUENCY: Repeat three times or alternately maintain the pose for one or two minutes as convenient with normal, slow rhythmic breathing.

FOR THE BEGINNERS:

(v) If Padmasana is difficult, do it in Sukhasana or loosen the foot-lock in Padmasana but keep the knees as near the floor as possible.

(vi) CONTRA-INDICATED: During the first 3 days of menstruation and last few months of pregnancy.

(vii) BENEFITS: It normalises uterine functioning in case of women, promotes health of the deeper sex organs with the pelvis and the ovaries; provides internal massage to the various endocrine glands; tones up the lungs and muscles of the chest; by checking the free circulation of blood to the extremities, the trunk derives an increased supply of blood; tones up the abdominal viscera and reduces excess fat in the abdomen; helps diabetics with improvement in general metabolism.

4.4.4 Shalabhasana (*Locust Pose*)

(i) POSTURE: Lie flat on your abdomen, arms on the respective sides. Inhale. Raise backward both the legs together with exhalation but without raising the head.

(ii) METHOD: *First variation* (alternate use of leg)

1. Lie down with face downwards and chin on the floor with feet together and soles turned upwards.
2. Stretch the arms along the sides and clench your fists and inhale or keep the hands under the thighs (Fig. 19a).

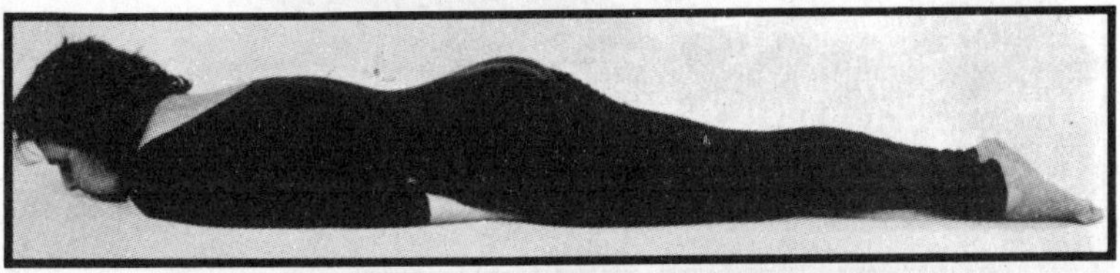

3. Raise right leg as high as you can with exhalation, putting up mild pressure on the clenched fists (Fig. 19b). Don't

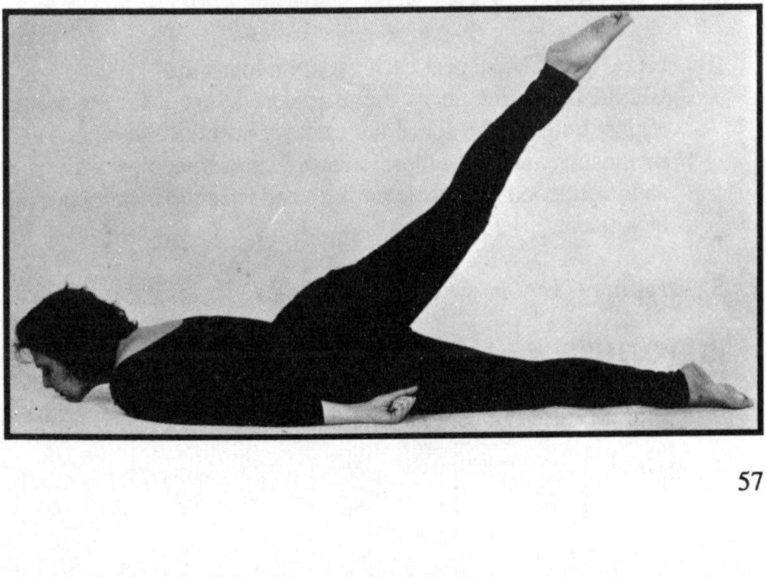

raise the head or bend the knees.

4. Lower the leg slowly to the floor with inhalation and relax.

Second Variation

5. Keep your palms underneath the upper portion of the thighs and inhale.
6. Raise both the legs together as high as possible with exhalation (Fig. 19c).

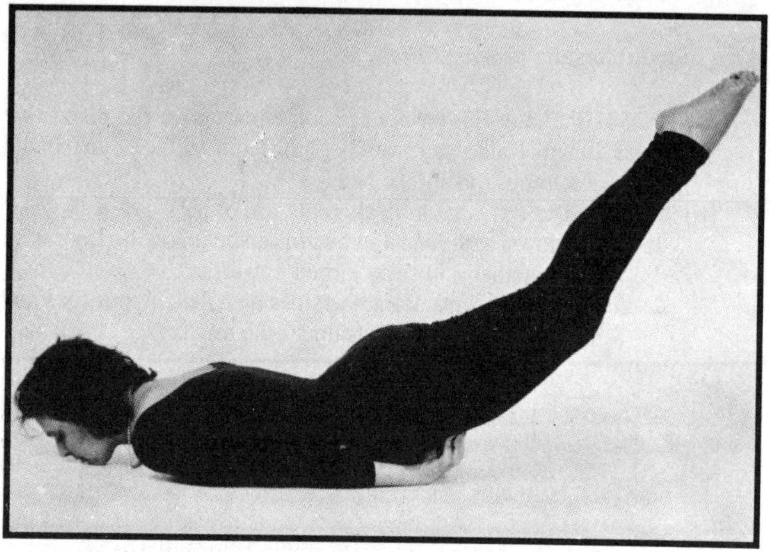

7. Slowly lower the legs, with inhalation, and relax.

(iii) RHYTHM: EXH SUS INH
3 : 6 : 3

(iv) FREQUENCY: Repeat each variation four times.

(v) BENEFITS: Strengthens the leg muscles; exercises the pelvic region; tones up the dorsal muscles and benefits in lumbago and rheumatic pains in the hips; reduces fatness from hips, waist and abdomen; good for dysmenorrhoea and irregular menses in case of women.

4.4.5 Ustrasana (*The Camel Pose*) - For women

(i) POSTURE: With knees and toes touching the ground, kneel down and bend your head and waist backwards while breathing in and hold the raised heels with your hands.

Note: To be practised much later, when other exercises are successfully performed.

(ii) METHOD

1. Assume sitting posture as in kneeling (Fig. 20a). Support the body on the toes and the knees and gradually lean backwards.

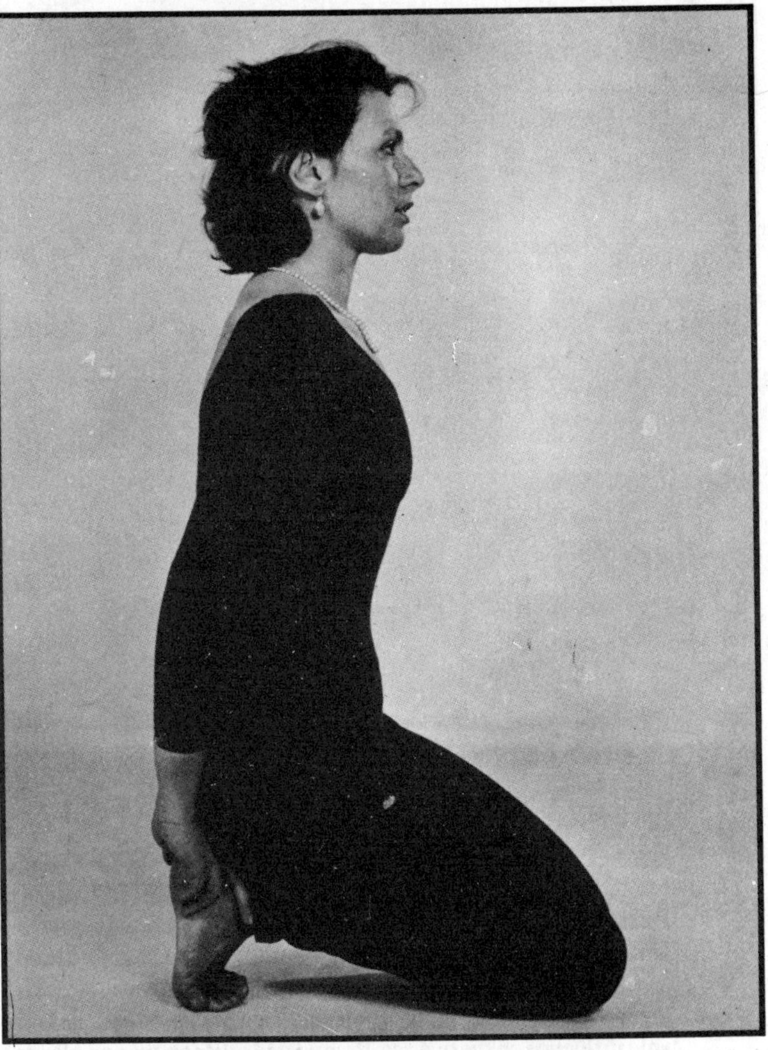

2. Fix the arms from behind and put them on heels - fingers pointing outwards and the thumbs towards the toes.

3. Keep the arms straight, slowly lift the pelvis while taking the breath in. Press the upper torso (body above the waist) slowly, both outward and upward, throwing the neck downward (Fig. 20b).

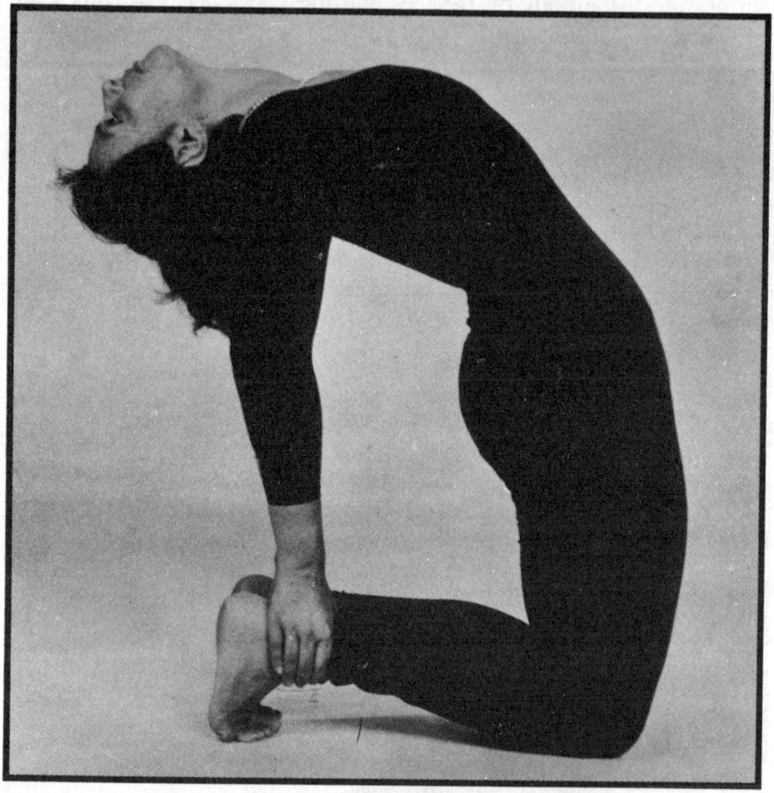

4. Return to kneeling position with exhalation.

(iii) RHYTHM: INH RET EXH

3 : 6 : 3

(iv) FREQUENCY: Repeat five times.

(v) BENEFITS: Anterior stretch of the spine; prevents flabbiness and relieves vertebral pressure; promotes spinal circulation; strengthens urogenital muscles; exercises all the deep muscles of the inner side of the thighs, trunk and the neck; produces favourable influence on the ovaries, thyroid and other endocrine glands.

4.4.6 Dhanurasana (*The bow-curve Pose*)

(i) POSTURE: Lie on your chest and abdomen. Hold both the ankles with the respective hands and exert pressure to raise your head and chest, the knees and legs from the ground, while breathing in.

Initial state to Learn

Variation I - Naukasana Type (the boat pose)

(ii) METHOD

1. With your arms behind the back or palms under the thing, raise simultaneously the head, the chest and the legs from the ground, with inhalation.
2. Try to raise it equal on both sides.
3. Repeat three or four times.

Variation II

1. Bend legs at the knees, raise the head and chest.
2. Catch hold of the legs firmly at the ankles with the respective hands (Fig. 21a).

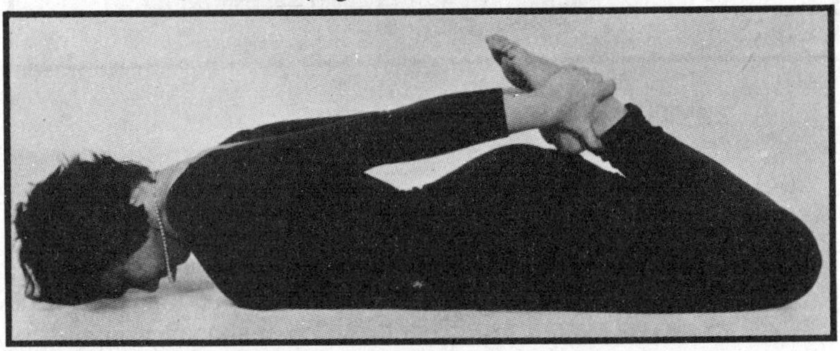

3. Pull upwards on the ankles while inhaling, lifting the thighs off the floor. Only abdomen and pelvis remain in contact with the floor and the spine looks like a stretched bow (Fig. 21b).
4. Try to keep the knees together and retain the pose for six seconds.
5. Release the hold on the ankles with exhalation and stretch fully the legs. Beginners can keep their knees spread apart but the feet to be kept together on an equal level. This will help you to raise the thighs more easily.

Note: **If it is difficult, practise the I variation only as mentioned above. Those who have a weak abdomen should not do this practice.**

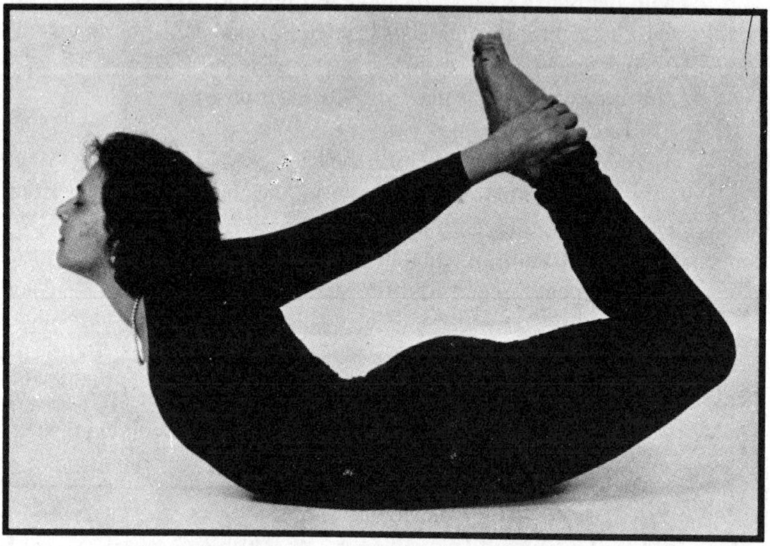

(iii) RHYTHM: INH RET EXH
3 : 6 : 3

(iv) FREQUENCY: Repeat five times. Pause or relax after each round.

(v) BENEFITS: Anterior stretch throughout the spinal column; extraordinary intra-abdominal pressure; fresh supply of blood to the abdominal viscera, especially to the lower abdomen and the sex organs; gives exercise to neck, arms and shoulders; healthy effect on the prostate gland and kidneys; good exercise to the arms, shoulders, neck, back, legs and ankles; stimulates pancreatic action in diabetics.

4.5 SPINAL TWIST

4.5.1 Vakrasana (*Twist of the spine*)

(i) POSTURE: Sit with legs stretched forward. With arms thrown in front, rotate sidewards alternately while exhaling.

(ii) METHOD

1. Sit with legs stretched forward, touching each other.
2. Throw arms in front, parallel to the floor, palms downward - inhale (Fig. 22a).

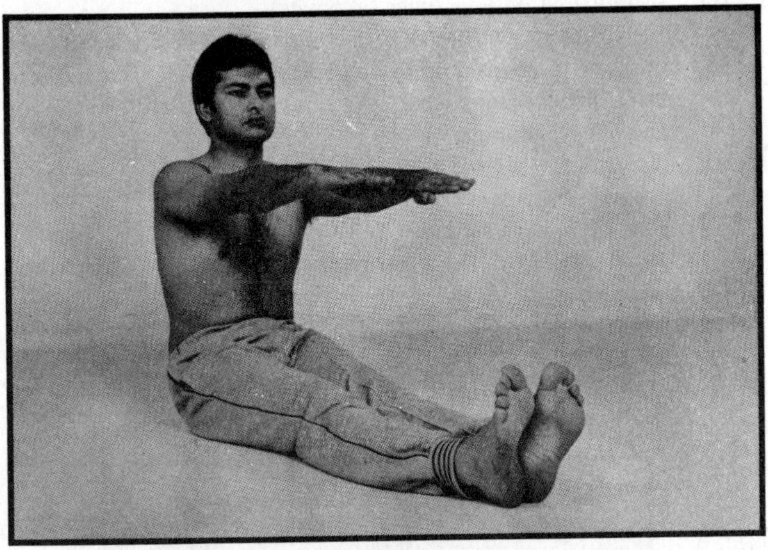

3. Rotate sidewards along with the arms, while you exhale (Fig. 22b).

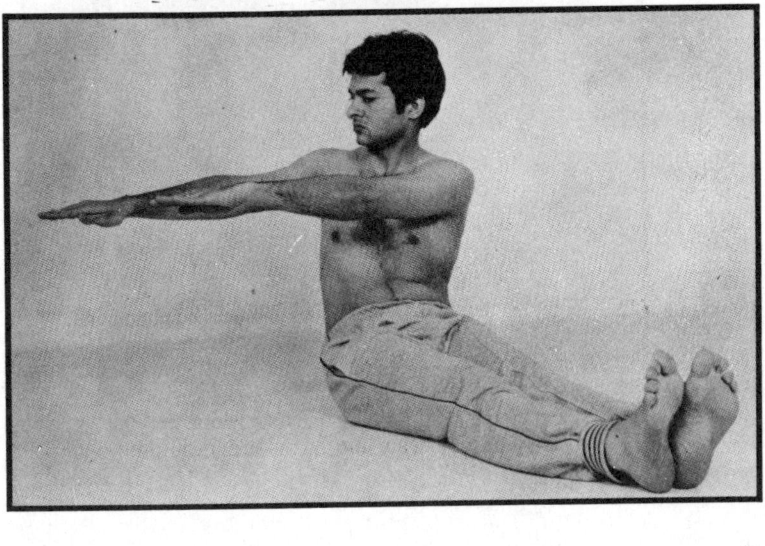

4. Return to starting position while you inhale.
5. Repeat on the other side.

(iii) RHYTHM: EXH INH
3 : 3

(iv) FREQUENCY: Five times (alternate).

(v) BENEFITS: Gentle twist of spine; removes obesity; removal of minor displacements of vertebrae; removal of lateral curvature of spine; prepares for advance practices like Konasana III variation and Matsyendrasana.

4.5.2 Konasana (*The Angle Pose*) - Variation III

Twisting the spine standing

(i) POSTURE: With feet apart and arms spread out in a standing position, try to touch the big toe with opposite hand alternately while breathing out.

(ii) METHOD

1. Stand with feet 24" apart, feet in the same line. Stretch out arms to sides, palms up and open.

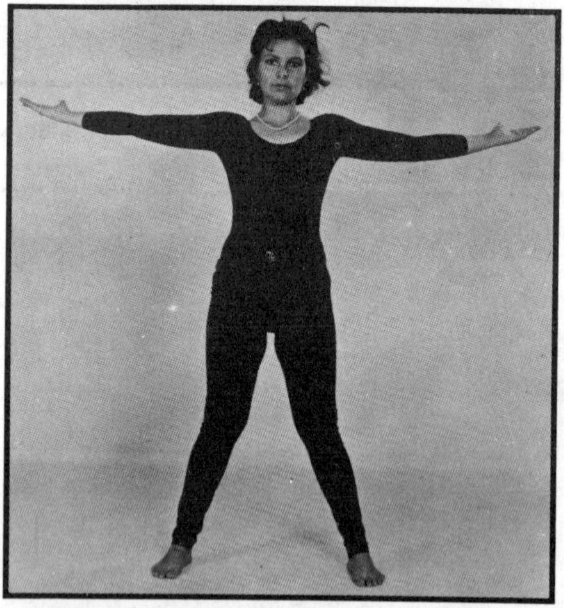

2. While inhaling, draw the arms and shoulders backward (Fig. 23a).

3. Bend forward, sideways with exhalation, turning the body above waist to left side, trying to touch the left toe with right hand (Fig. 23b).

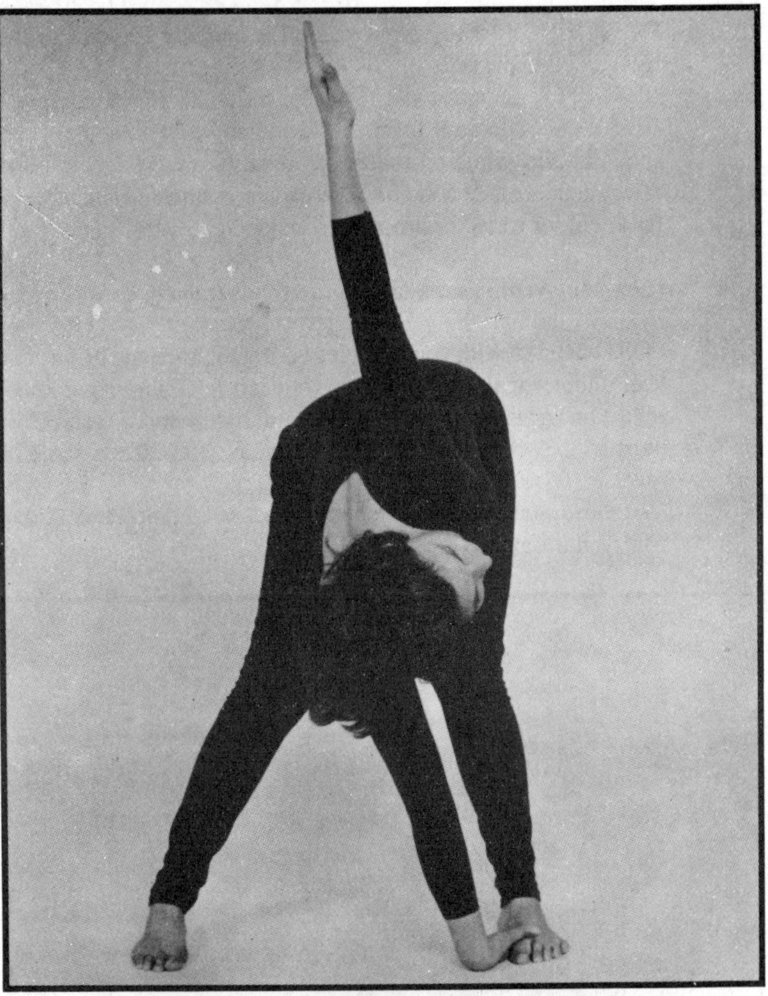

4. No bending of legs, and hips to remain in normal position.
5. Turn the neck left and upwards and try to look up at the left palm which is stretched up.
6. Maintain the pose for six seconds in suspension.
7. Return to normal position while inhaling, with arms stretched out.

8. Repeat on the other side, trying to touch the right tow with the left hand.

(iii) RHYTHM: EXH SUS INH
3 : 6 : 3

(iv) FREQUENCY: Three times alternate bending forward to the right and the left side.

(v) BENEFITS: Lateral twist to spine; intra-abdominal compression; reduces fatness from the abdomen; exercises the neck, shoulder and arms; promotes oxygenation of the lungs; good effect in the case of abdominal disorders, contracted chest, weak back and for round or drooping shoulders.

4.5.3 Ardha-Matsyendrasana (*Semi Matsyendrasana*)

(i) POSTURE: Sit with your right leg bent at the knee and bring your heel under left thigh. Interlock your left heel with right knee. Inhale and grasp your left big tow with right-hand fingers. Give twist to the whole trunk with exhalation. Repeat the same in reverse.

First variation: For the Beginners: - Practise Incomplete or Ardha Matsyendrasana.

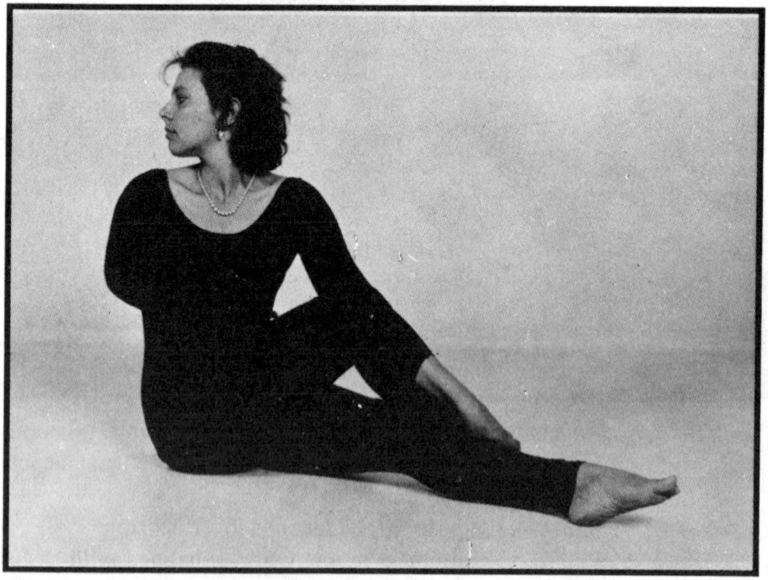

(ii) METHOD

1. Sit on the ground and spread the left leg in front.
2. Place the right foot on the side of your left knee.
3. Breathe in.
4. Pass your left arm around the right knee and hold your foot with your left hand. Take your right hand behind your back.
5. Turn the head and the trunk to your right as far as it can go, with exhalation, and tilt the turned head downwards - do not let the knee of the left leg rise from the ground (Fig. 24a).
6. Hold for 6 seconds in a period of suspension.
7. Release your hands and unwind the trunk, breathing in.
8. Repeat the same with the right leg stretched and putting the left foot beside the right knee.

(iii) RHYTHM: EXH SUS INH
3 : 6 : 3

(iv) FREQUENCY: Repeat three times.

Second Variation

(i) METHOD

1. Sit on the floor with both legs extended.
2. Fold the right leg and press the heel against the perineum or keep it near the anus.
3. Bring the left foot over the right knee and interlock it, place the sole of the foot on the floor - inhale.
4. Hold the toe of the left foot by right-hand fingers - left knee to come under the right armpit.
5. Swing the left arm from behind the back, palm outward.
6. While exhaling, twist the whole trunk towards the left side along with the head and shoulders (Fig. 24b).
7. Maintain pose during suspension for six seconds.
8. Twist the spine back to normal while breathing in.
9. Repeat, crossing the right foot over the left knee and twisting the spine to the right.

(ii) RHYTHM: EXH SUS INH
3 : 6 : 3

(iii) FREQUENCY: Four times alternate twist to right and left.

(iv) BENEFITS: Extreme left and right twist to the spine; helps in the removal of the lateral curvature of the spine; increases venous circulation in the abdominal zone; tones up liver, spleen and pancreas; good for maintaining tone and pliancy of spine; good in case of sexual debility; promotes gastric secretions and improves appetite; good for those suffering from stiff neck, lumbago and rheumatism of the back muscles; effective in dyspepsia, asthma and diabetes.

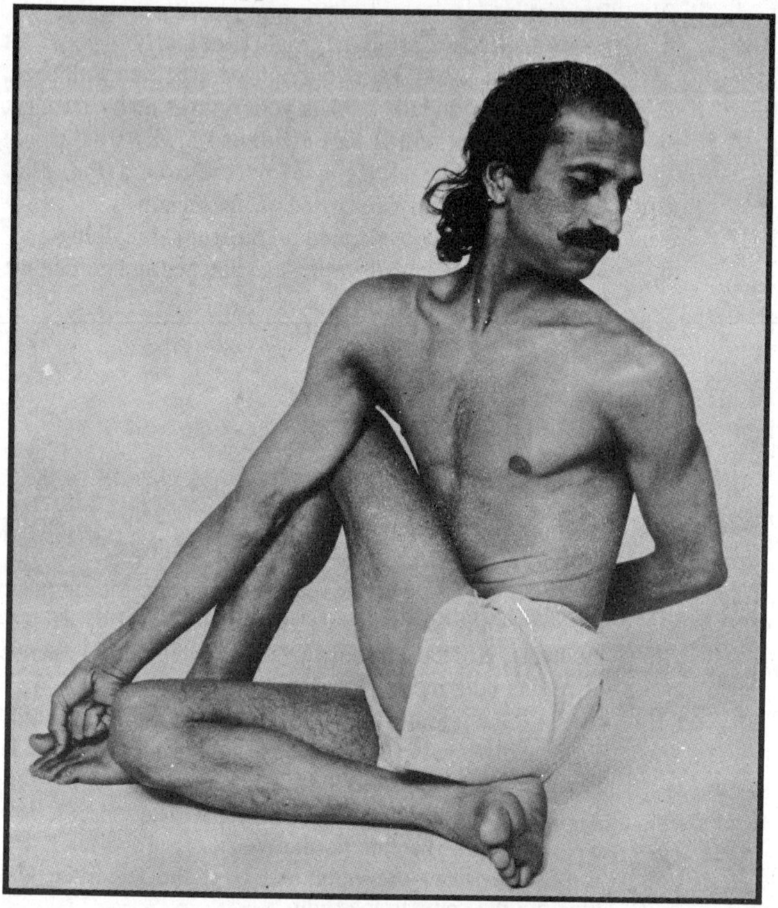

Note: People with weak abdominal wall and hernia trouble should avoid this asana.

5

EXERCISES FOR THE ABDOMEN

5.1 YOGA MUDRA (*The Symbol of Yoga*)

5.1.1 Yoga Mudra in Sukhasana – Easy for the beginners –Refer 4.3.1.

5.1.2 Yoga Mudra in Padmasana

When you have learnt Padmasana, you can try Yoga Mudra in Padmasana where the intra-abdominal compression is much increased.

(i) METHOD

1. Form the foot-lock in Padmasana and adjust your heels comfortably pressing them (the heels) firmly against the upper front margin of the pubic bone (above the sex organ).
2. Hold the wrist of one hand with the other, at the back.
3. With exhalation, bend the head and trunk towards the knees alternately, coming to the upright seated position every time while inhaling (Fig. 25a).

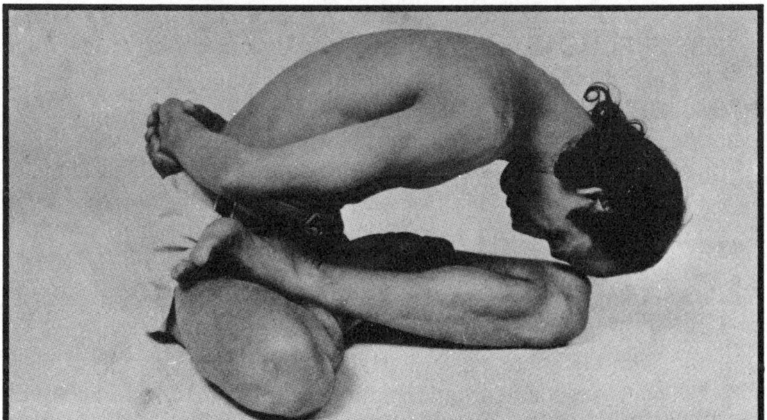

4. Then bend forward in the centre with the exhalation – Does your head reach the floor? With practice, gradually it will – never force yourself to touch the floor (Fig. 25b).
5. Come back to the starting upright position, inhaling.

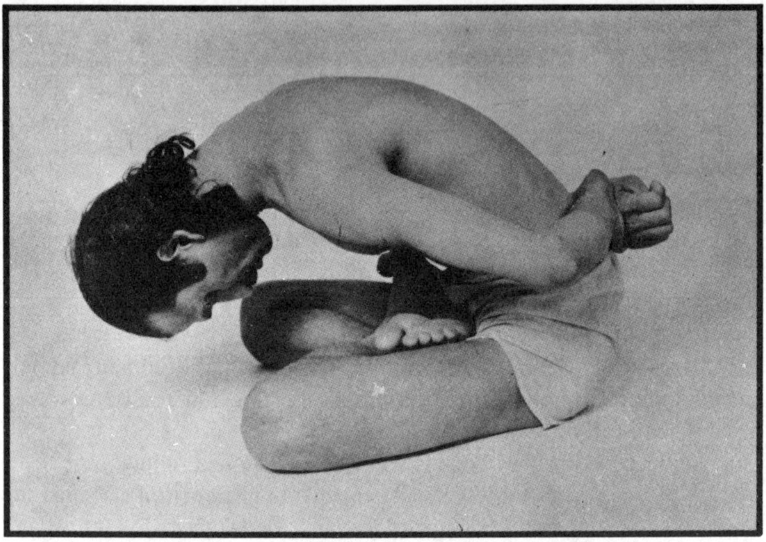

Note: See that the spine is arched in forward bending position.

(ii) RHYTHM: EXH SUS INH
3 : 6 : 3

(iii) FREQUENCY: Three rounds (bending alternately to both the knees and the centre is one round).

(iv) BENEFITS: Increases intra-abdominal compression; restores abdominal viscera (organs) to their proper places. Tones up and gives massage to small intestine, colon, prostate and kidneys. Strengthens the muscular wall of the abdomen. Provides relief in chronic constipation and helps in peristalsis.

5.2. PAVANMUKTASANA (*The Anti-flatus Pose or Gas-release Pose*)

(i) POSTURE: Folding the leg (alternately) or both the legs together over the abdomen while breathing out and pressing the knee with your hands.

(ii) METHOD

Variation I: One-leg anti-flatus pose (Ekapada type)

1. Lie supine at full length, arms on sides, inhale.
2. Lift one leg, fold at the knee-point while exhaling and hold it by clasping both hands, fingers interlocking.
3. Press the knee on the stomach, the other leg to be kept straight on the floor (Fig. 26a).
4. Retain the posture for four seconds in suspension with the pressing of the knee.

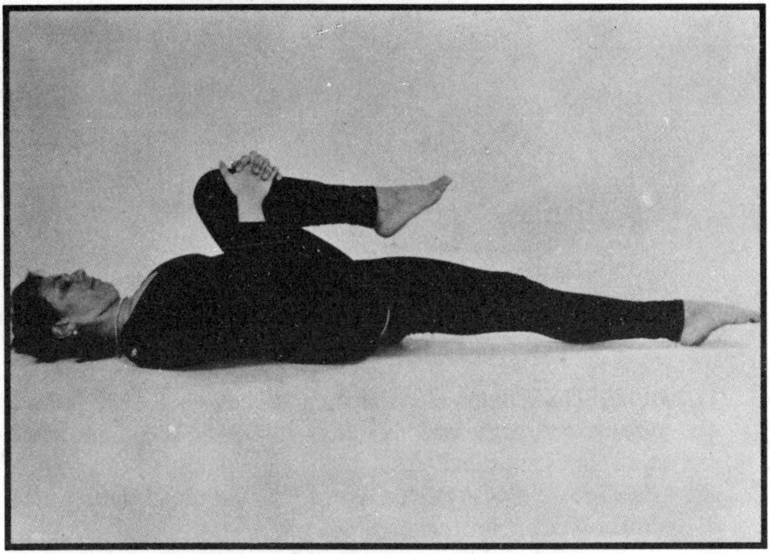

5. Return to normal position while inhaling.
6. Repeat with the other leg.

(iii) RHYTHM: EXH SUS INH

2 : 4 : 2

(iv) FREQUENCY: Four times alternately with each leg.

Variation II: Both the legs anti-flatus pose (Dwipada type).

(v) METHOD:

1. The technique is the same as in Ekapada, but in this variation, fold both the legs at the knee joints together and fold your arms around the folded legs.
2. Maintain the posture with knees pressed against the chest in a period of suspension of the breath (Fig. 26b).

3. Knees and feet to remain together.
4. Release both the legs with inhalation and rest before repeating the round.

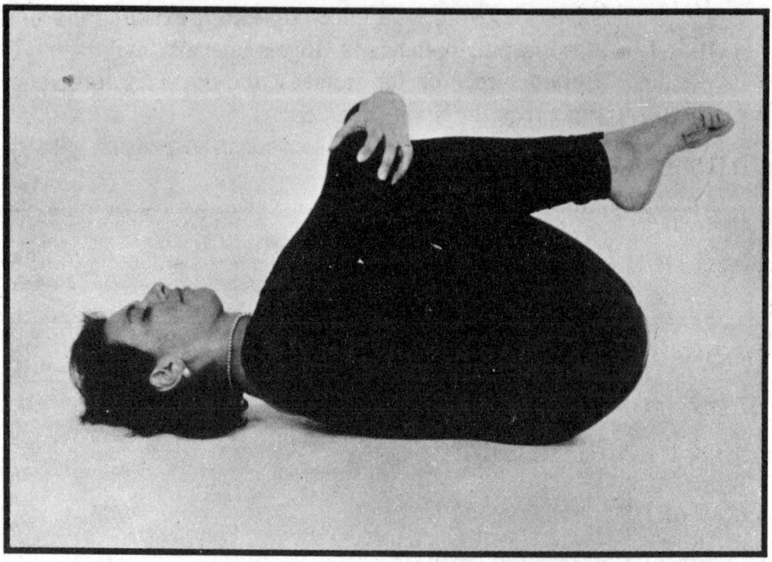

(vi) BENEFITS: Compresses abdomen and helps in the expulsion of gases; exercises the various joints — hip-joint, knee-joint, ankle-joint. Cures constipation.

(vii) CONTRA-INDICATED: Women should avoid during menstruation and in pregnancy.

5.3 HASTAPADANGUSTASANA (*The Toe-Finger Pose*)

The Dynamic Type — Three variations

(i) POSTURE: In standing position with legs together, throw right leg and left leg forward alternately, with exhalation, and then sidewards and backwards — trunk to be kept straight.

(ii) METHOD: *Variation I*

1. Stand with legs together.
2. Raise right hand forward, palm down, inhale.
3. Throw right leg forward, exhaling, keeping left arm on side — body should be kept straight and do not bend the leg (Fig. 27a).

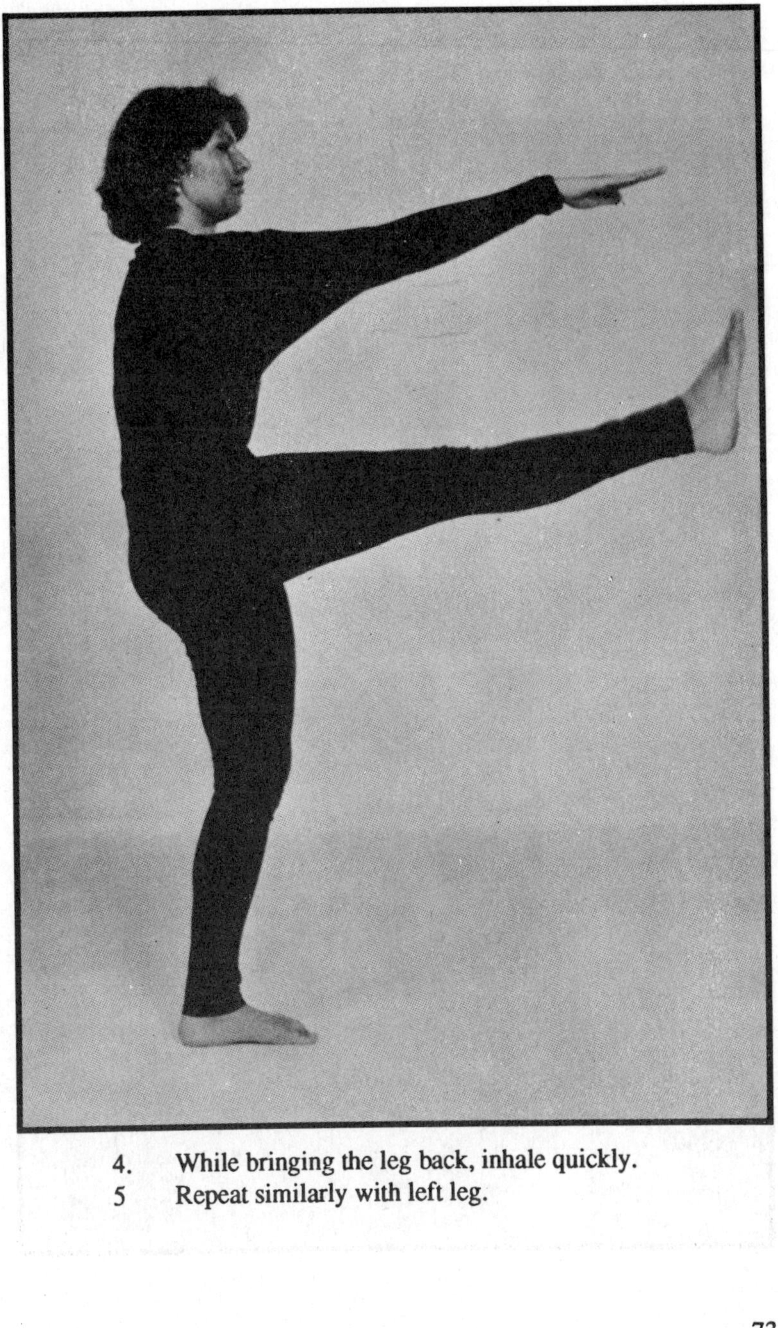

4. While bringing the leg back, inhale quickly.
5 Repeat similarly with left leg.

Variation II

In this variation, throw the leg sidewards alternately, keeping hands on the waist (Fig. 27b).

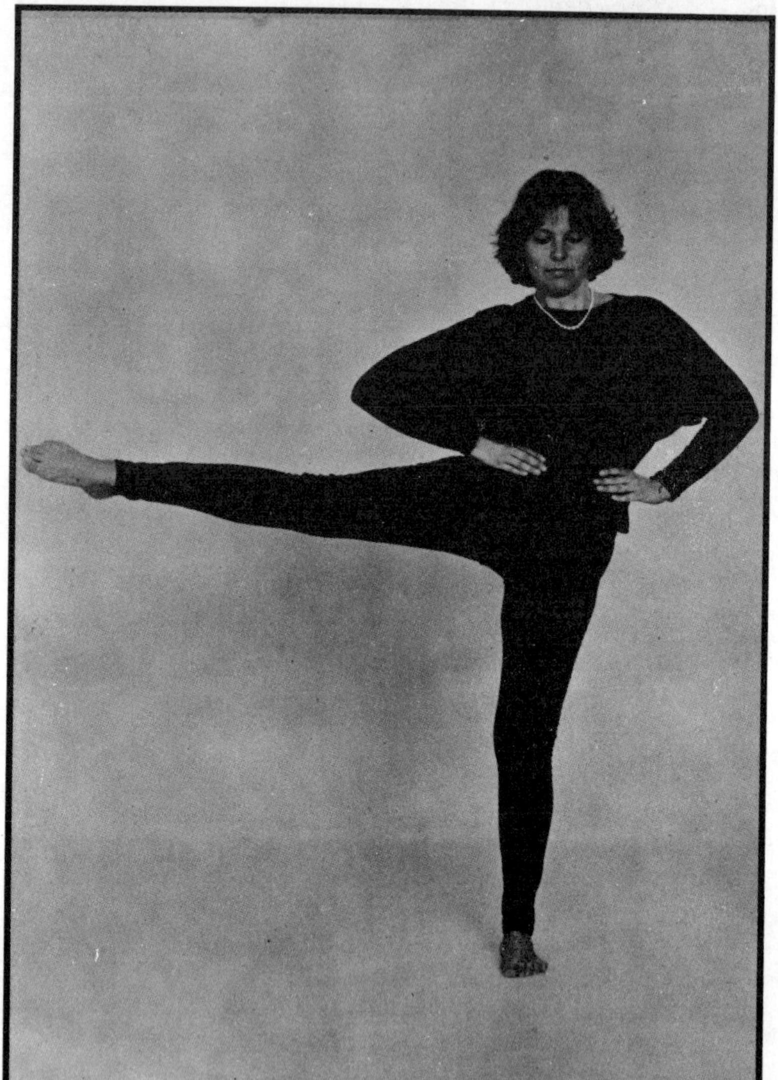

Vatiation III

In this variation, throw the leg backwards alternately with hands on waist, thumb touching the spine at the back (Fig. 27c).

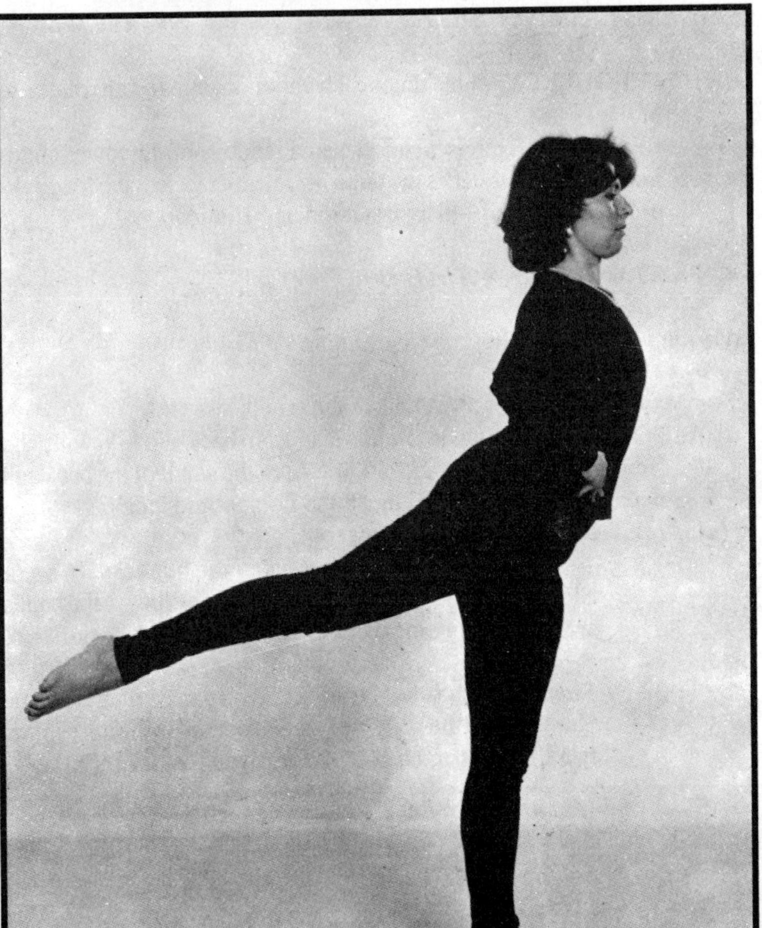

Note: You have to exhale and inhale quickly whiledoing the leg mevement. Keep the leg straight as far as possible and the body erect with no bending.

(iii) RHYTHM: EXH INH
3 : 3

(iv) FREQUENCY: Three times each variation, making alternate use of leg.

(v) BENEFITS: Exercises muscles and tendons of the lower abdomen and hips; stretches the thigh muscles; exercises the lower extremities and helps in assimilation and elimination.

5.4 PARYANKASANA (*The Hamsa Pose*)

Variation I: Supta Vajrasana (*The Supine Vajrasana*)

For flexion of the knees and to make the thighs less tense.

(i) POSTURE: Sitting in Vajrasana, lean back slowly with the support of your hands and elbows. Arch the small of the back and make the top of the head touch the floor, while inhaling.

(ii) METHOD:

1. Assume Vajrasana with feet under the buttocks.
2. Slowly lean backward with the aid of the elbows and hands while breathing in, keeping the knees, as far as possible, together.
3. Stretch your head as far back as you can so that the spine is arched and the body weight is taken up by the top of your head, elbows and hands, the legs and feet (Fig. 28a).

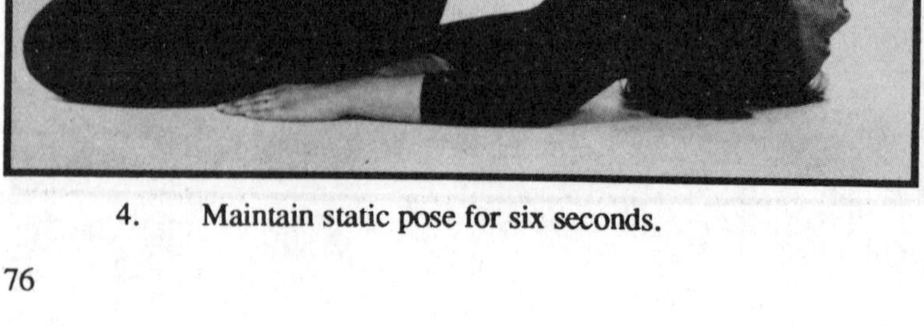

4. Maintain static pose for six seconds.

5. To return, widen the knees and simultaneously hold the ankles firmly with your hands, return to the Vajrasana position with exhalation.

(iii) RHYTHM: INH RET EXH
4 : 6 : 4

(iv) FREQUENCY: Five times or do it once maintaining static pose for not more than two minutes with slow, normal rhythmic abdominal breathing.

Precautions

a) Bend backward in stages, taking the help of your elbows one after the other.

b) If thighs become too tense and painful, widen the distance between the knees. When the posture is perfected, bring them closer and do not lift the knees.

c) For coming to the starting position, raise trunk and head off the floor first with the help of your elbows.

Variation II: **Paryankasana** (*the final position*)

Head and shoulders should touch the ground and the entire back should be as much in contact with the ground as possible (flat). Either interlace the fingers and hold the hands over the chest or one can fold the arms at the elbow joint and make it serve as a cushion to rest the back of the head (Fig. 28b).

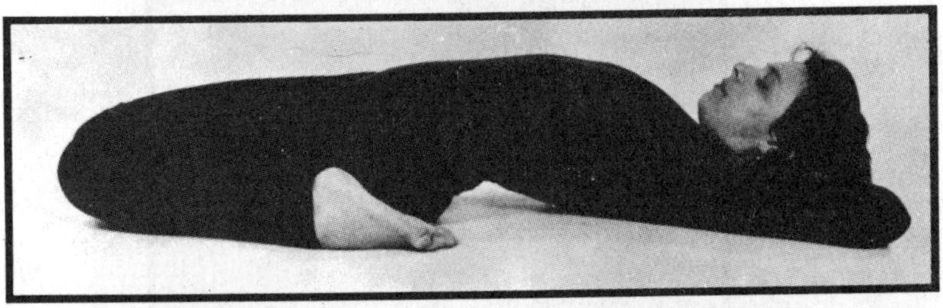

(vii) BENEFITS: Full stretching of the abdominal and pelvic muscles and muscles on the inner side of the thigh; deep pressure on the utero-abdominal and genito-urinary organs. Great value for women during pregnancy and for painless childbirth.

(viii) CONTRA-INDICATED: Discontinue during pregnancy and first three days of menstruation. In the beginning, try flexion of the knees only.

5.5 HASTAPADASANA (*Arm-leg Pose*)

Refer Section 4.3.

6

EXERCISES FOR EXTREMITIES

6.1 UTKATASANA (*The Semi-standing Pose*)

(i) POSTURE: Standing in Talasana position with feet apart raise your heels and squat slowly while breathing out.

(ii) METHOD

1. Stand in Talasana position. Inhale and rise on toes, raising arms parallel to the ground. (Fig. 29a).

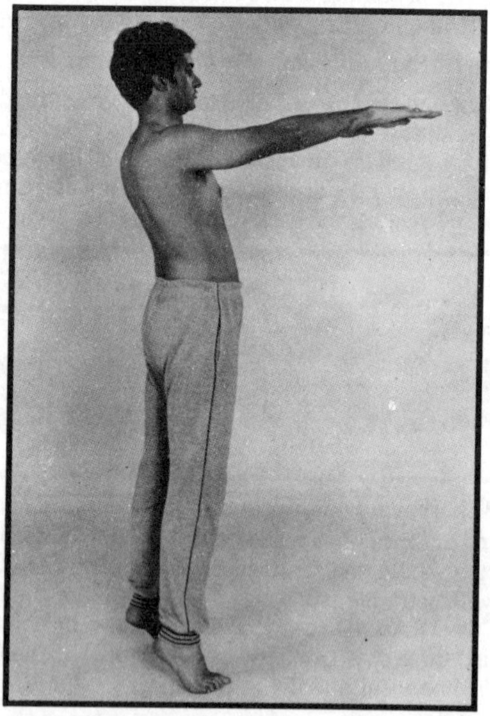

2. Hold breath for four seconds.
3. Squat slowly while exhaling — chest erect.

4. Remain for four seconds without breath — buttocks resting on heels, thighs a little apart (Fig. 29b).
5. Return to the starting position, slowly inhaling.

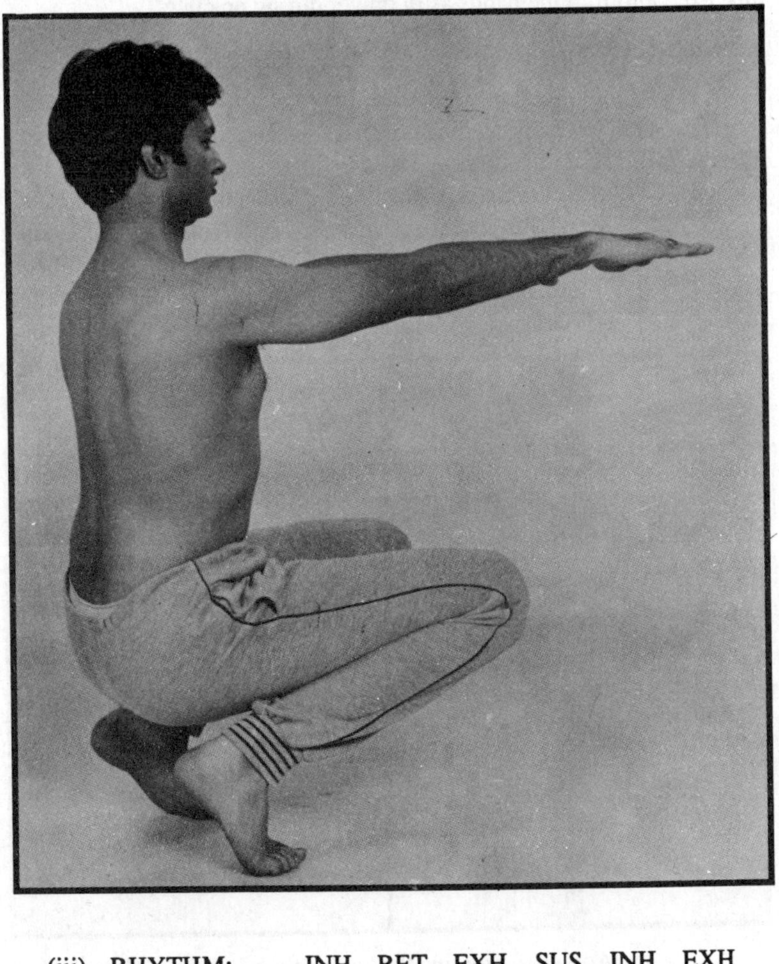

(iii) RHYTHM:

INH	RET	EXH	SUS	INH	EXH
2 :	4 :	2 :	4 :	2 :	2

(iv) FREQUENCY: Six times.

(v) BENEFITS: Exercises the muscles of the leg (thigh and calf); provides abdominal compression specially to pelvic area. Provides coordination and balance.

6.2 NATA PRARTHANASANA: (*For women*)

Method and benefits of Nata Prarthanasana are the same as in Utkatasana, except to fold the hands as in prayer during practice.

6.3 EK-PADASANA (The One-leg Pose) or (Vrikshasana)

(i) POSTURE: In standing position to balance on one leg alternately.

(ii) METHOD

1. Stand relaxed in prayer pose with both legs together.
2. Bend, lift your right leg and place its sole against the inner part of your left thigh (Fig. 30a).
3. Maintain balance and stand on the left leg — take aid if necessary.

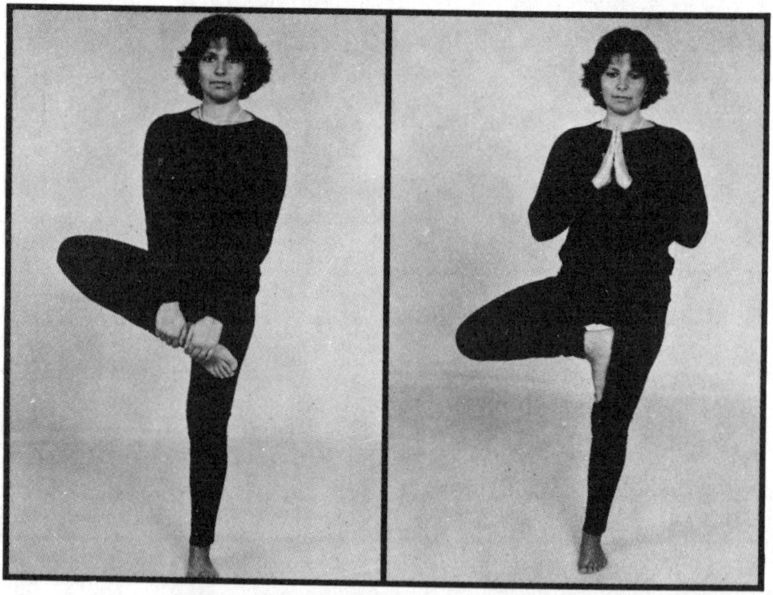

4. Adjust by pressing the heel of the raised leg tightly against the opposite groin — sole against the opposite thigh.
5. After you have achieved balance by practice, arrange the hands in prayer form (folded). (Fig. 30b).
6. Close your eyes and try to keep still and motionless. Concentrate on body movements and check them.
7. Do it with the other leg.

(iii) RHYTHM: Normal breathing.

(iv) FREQUENCY: Maintain the pose for a few seconds and gradually increase it to two minutes — three times alternately with each leg.

(v) BENEFITS: Exercises and alternately relaxes the muscles of the leg; promotes neuro-muscular co-ordination and balance. Increases endurance; helps to gain nerve control and steadiness.

6.4 BHADRASANA (*The Throne Pose or Good Pose*)

The easy one

(i) POSTURE: In a sitting position, fold both legs inwards with soles together. Draw feet close to your body while breathing in.

(ii) METHOD

1. Sit with legs fully stretched out.
2. Fold both legs simultaneously, soles of the feet touching each other. Hold the feet with both hands and draw them nearer the body so that heels are placed below the genitals. Inhale during the process (Fig. 31).

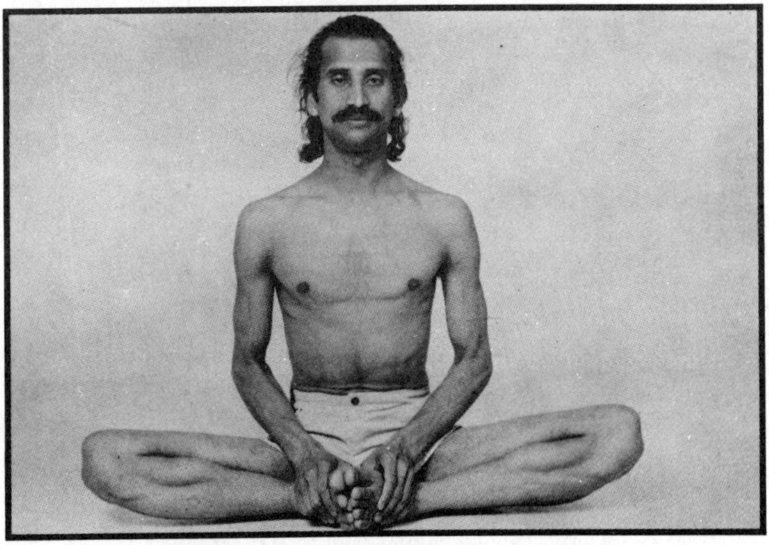

3. Give a little swing when you press the knees to touch the floor, keep the upper part of the body and neck erect, as far as possible.

4. Place the hands, if you can, on respective knees, pressing them down but maintain toes together, otherwise hold the toes with hands.
5. While exhaling, throw the legs together forward.
6. Repeat without pause.

(iii) RHYTHM:

INH		RET		EXH
3	:	10	:	2

(iv) FREQUENCY: Four times.

(v) BENEFITS: Exercises both the superficial and deep muscles of the inner side of thigh; strengthens muscles and ligaments of the urogenital region; helps when troubled by night emission. Favourably effects the pelvic organs, the groin, the thighs and sex organ.

Note : If your knees do not touch the floor — swing your knees up and down but do not bend forward. With sufficient practice, thighs and knees will lower themselves and rest on the floor.

6.5 HASTAPADANGUSTASANA (*The Toe-finger Pose*)

The Dynamic Variations — Refer Section 5.3

7

HEAD-LOW POSTURES

7.1 SARVANGASANA (*All-body-reverse Pose*) A Static Pose

(i) POSTURE: Lie on your back — raise legs pushing up the hips and supporting your trunk with your palms. Make the legs straight and maintain the pose with slow breathing.

(ii) METHOD

1. Initially start with Andhra-Sarvangasana or the Semi-reverse pose.
2. Lie supine, body at full length, arms on respective sides, take a deep breath.
3. Fold the legs, slowly exhale and with a little jerk, raise the lower part of the body, pushing up from buttocks and hold the waist with hands.
4. Balance entire body-weight upon the palms, the elbows, the neck and back of the head.
5. Fold the legs at the knee or raise the legs, whatever is convenient and easily manageable.
6. Maintain the pose with slow, normal rhythmic breathing for not more than two minutes.
7. Slowly come back to the starting position with inhalation.

(iii) SPECIAL INSTRUCTIONS: Do not repeat. In the beginning start the asana with 30 seconds of static position and gradually increase the duration to a maximum of three minutes. Do not get up immediately — adequate rest at least for two minutes, should follow. Best done on empty stomach.

(iv) CAUTION: Those suffering from eye trouble, high blood pressure or heart trouble should not try this asana. Women should discontinue during menstruation or pregnancy.

(v) SARVANGASANA : The complete all-body-reverse pose: After three weeks, go in for Sarvangasana. Raise the legs up and try to make the body straight as much as possible, making a right angle, and the body weight almost shifting to neck and back of the head. Maintain this static position for a maximum of three minutes (Fig. 32).

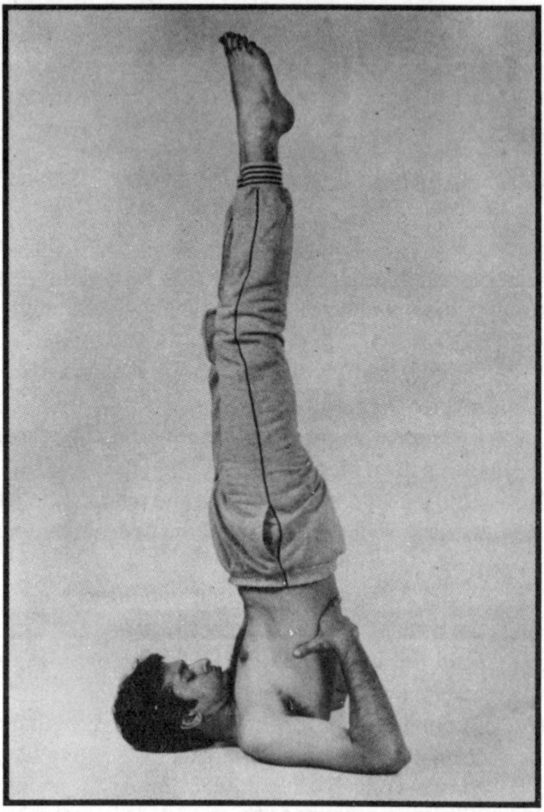

(vi) BENEFITS: Only practice that improves circulation in brain; affects favourably the glandular system especially the thyroid; brings relief from congestion in the abdominal and pelvic regions; helps in general and sexual debility; good for those suffering from ailments like constipation, dyspepsia, headache, neurasthenia, etc. Prevents the ptosis or prolapse of the uterus. Provides relief in varicose veins in the legs.

Note : Practice of Sarvangasana will be easier if Vipritkarni is perfected first.

7.2 VIPARITAKARNI (*Inverted Balance*)

A Static Pose — Recommended for women

(i) POSTURE: It is like Sarvangasana but in this posture the trunk is kept in a slanting position and not perpendicular to the floor.

(ii) METHOD:

1. Lie supine, body at full length, arms on respective sides.
2. Assume the semi-reverse pose of Ardha-Sarvangasana.
3. Slowly raise the legs high up perpendicular and keep the trunk in a slanting position — the back and the neck well-rested on the ground.
4. Carefully shift your hands slowly from the hips to the waist and adjust the grip so that you can hold the trunk properly (Fig. 33).

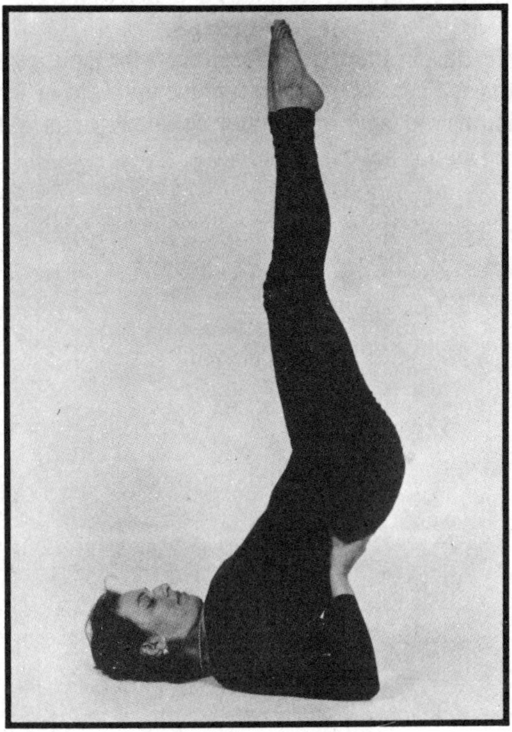

5. Maintain pose for a maximum of two minutes with abdominal breathing. While inhaling, return to starting position.
6. Do not repeat.

(iii) SPECIAL INSTRUCTIONS: Same as in Sarvangasana

(iv) CAUTION: As in Sarvangasana, during advanced pregnancy, its practice should be discontinued.

(v) RHYTHM: Normal breathing (abdominal)

(vi) FREQUENCY: Only once — maximum 2 minutes.

(vii) BENEFITS: Psycho-physical and neuro-muscular practice with many physiologic advantages; process aids digestion; increases supply of blood to the thorax and the head; promotes health of the sex organs; causes increase of blood pressure, pulse and respiration; good for those suffering from cerebral anaemia, sexual debility, prolapse of the uterus and congestion etc.

Note: Viparitakarni and Sarvangasana give the same results and benefits as Sirshasana. The technique involved in Sirshasana has intrinsic danger and would definitely harm old people for whom it is not recommended.

8

UNDERSTANDING OF KRIYAS (Personal Hygiene)

8.1 INTRODUCTION

It was realized by the ancient yogis that physical activity alone through the process of asanas might not be sufficient to preserve good health. Care of the body-complex with its various parts, was needed to maintain high efficiency of work. Hence, HATHA YOGA develops a method of hygiene —cleanliness or shuddhi called ghatsya yoga or physiological yoga. There are six-fold purification processes (SAT-KARMA) according to the Yoga system of hygiene.

SAT-KARMA
(Six-fold purificatory process)

NETI	DHAUTI	BASTI	NAULI	KAPAL BHATI	TRATAK
Methods of nasal cleaning	Cleaning the alimentary canal	Cleaning the intestines	Abdominal massage	For sinuses	Care of the eyes

These kriyas, viz. neti, dhauti, basti, nauli, kapal bhati, and tratak are for the care of internal and external organs like ear, nose, eyes, sinuses, the food-tube, intestines etc. With the help of these kriyas, pathogenic metabolites (mul) are eliminated from the vital organs and the body is kept free from disease. There is a contrast between modern medical hygiene and ancient Yoga concept of good health. The former, which is negative, based on external aids to health, kills the carriers of disease, and the latter, a positive one, based on the inner health of all the vital organs strengthens one's own inherent vitality. It is a well-known physiological fact that no bacteria can thrive on an ideally healthy organism. Thus, maintenance of day-to-day good health is conducive to auto-immunization. This is made possible by a variety of anti-toxic measures and the daily practice of outer and inner cleanliness (mulasuddhi) of the body.

Some of these kriyas are very complicated and time-consuming and demand knowledge of proper and precise techniques. But a few simple kriyas can easily be integrated into your daily life and can serve as a useful and effective course of personal hygiene and preventive medicine with its therapeutic value as the best cure for certain diseases. Some simple practices for purification have been recommended in this book which can be safely practised by an average student. These kriyas pertain to teeth, tongue, nose, sinuses and eyes.

Remember, prevention is better than cure.

8.2 TRATAK: (*Central Fixation*)

(i) METHOD: For (a) The left shoulder gaze (*Vama Jatru Tratak*).
(b) The right shoulder gaze (*Dakshina Jatru Tratak*).

Sit in Sukhasana or Vajrasana. Keep the body erect, head steady, and neck straight. Keep the thumb in front of you and fix the eyes on the nail of your thumb. Slowly move the hand towards the end of your shoulder, keeping your eyes fixed on the thumb nail — eyes wide open — no turning of the head. Maintain the gaze without flickering eyelids (Fig. 34a). Repeat

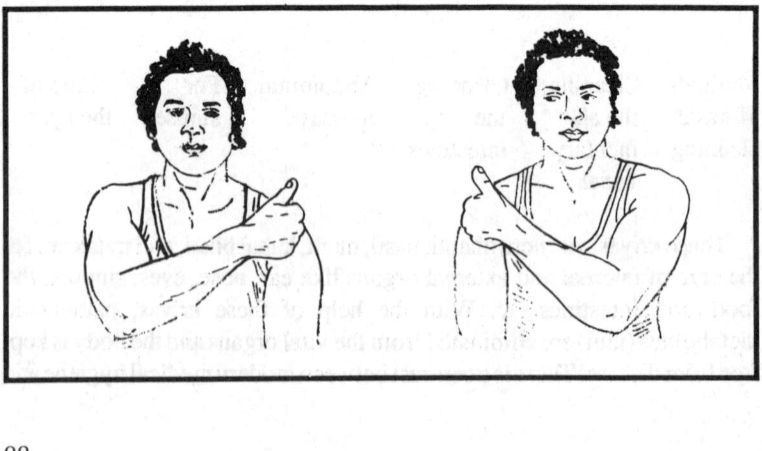

this for the other shoulder. Cup your hands and cover them over your closed eyes for rest, each time (Fig. 34b).

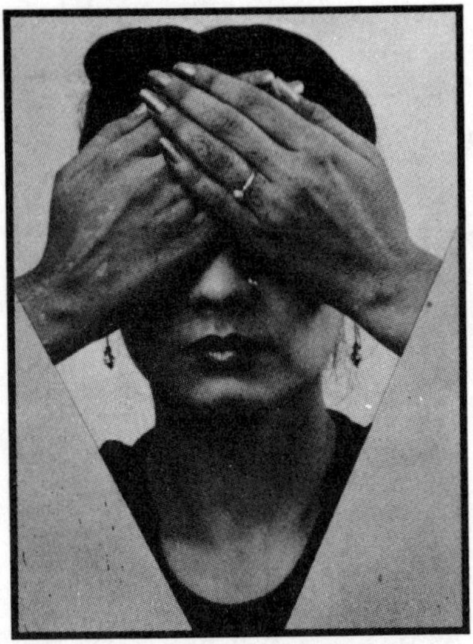

Note: Make use of the right thumb for left shoulder and the left thumb for the right shoulder. Women to use right thumb for right shoulder and left thumb for left shoulder for convenience.

(ii) RHYTHM: Normal breathing.

(iii) FREQUENCY: Three times (alternate) each shoulder gaze, increase duration from 15 seconds to one minute gradually.

(iv) BENEFITS: Exercise to the important eye muscles; improves minor eye defects; helps concentration; helps to secure proper fixation and accommodation.

(i) METHOD: For (c) the Nasal Gaze (Nasikagra) (Fig. 34d) (d) Space between the Eyebrows (Bhrumadhya) (Fig. 34e).

Sit in a comfortable meditative pose. Keeping eyes wide open, gaze at the tip of the nose without flickering eyelids. Now gaze at a point between the eyebrows similarly. If the eyes are tired, close them and cover with the palms of the hands. Alternately, do each gaze three times and increase the duration from 15 seconds to one minute.

(ii) BENEFITS: Same as mentioned above; helps in concentration.

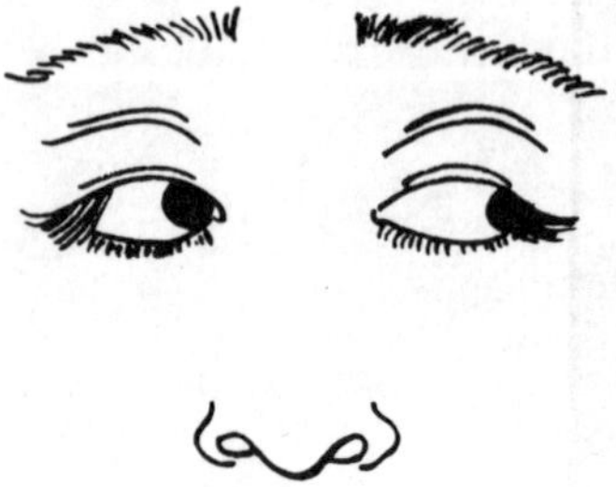

Fig. 34c
(a) VAMAJATRU

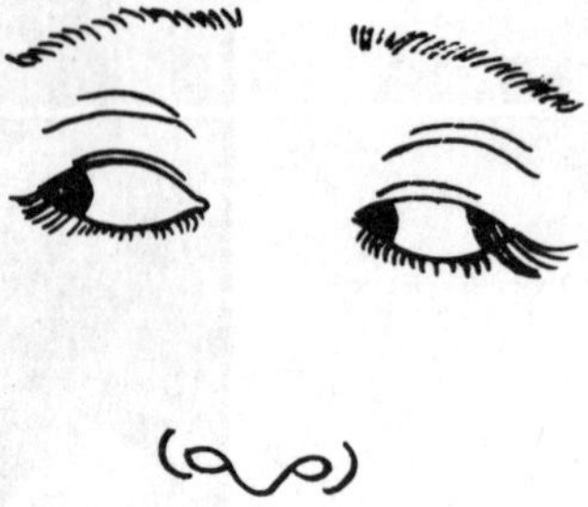

Fig. 34d
(b) DAKSINAJATRU

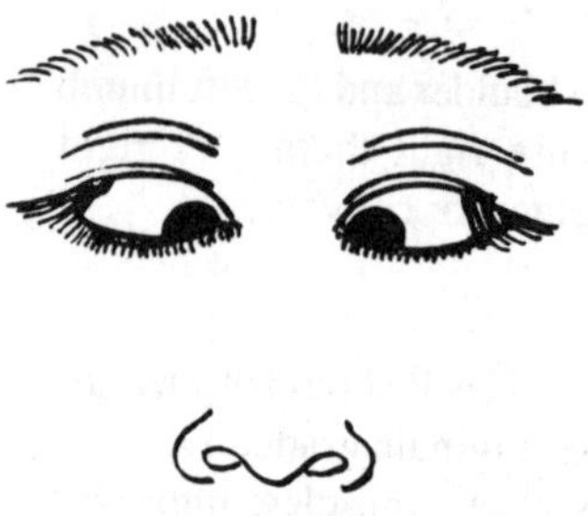

Fig. 34e
(c) NASIKAGRA

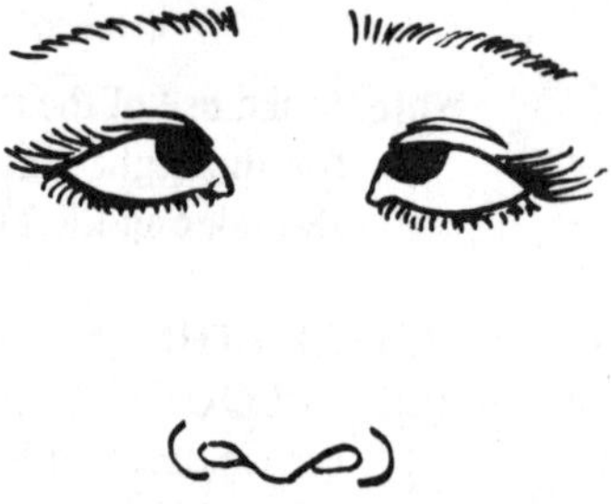

Fig 34f
(d) BHRUMADHYA

CARE OF THE EYES
Fig. 34c VAMA JATRU TRATAKA (Left shoulder gaze)
Fig. 34d DAKSINA JATRU TRATAKA (Right shoulder gaze)
Fig. 34e NASIKAGRA (the Nasal Gaze)
Fig. 34f Bhrumadhya (Space between the Eyebrows)

8.3 JALANETI (*Water Snuffing*)

(i) METHOD: Take a glassful of boiled water, put half a teaspoonful of table salt in it, stir it, let it cooled down to body temperature. Wash your hands with soap—do not use towel. Hold warm saline water in palm. Suck in water steadily with one nostril, closing the other with the forefinger of the other hand (Fig. 35). Manipulate and expel water from mouth. Blow your nostrils clear of all watery discharge. Repeat with the other nostril.

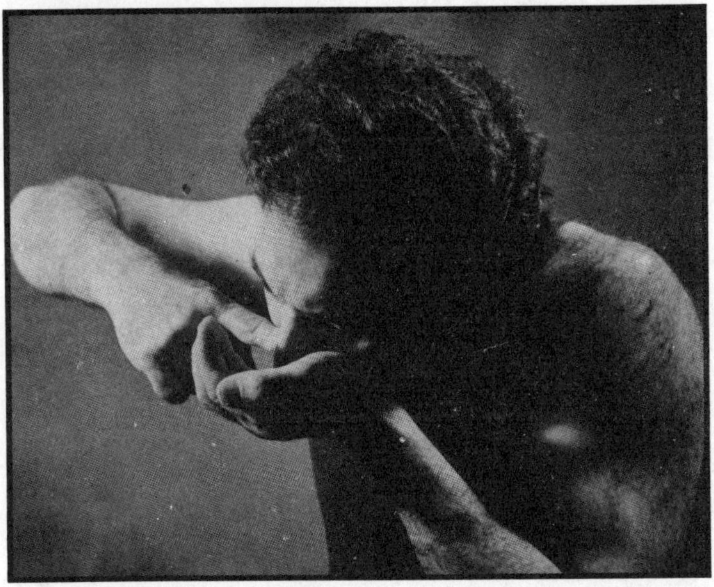

(ii) FREQUENCY: Only once with each nostril. Once or twice a week. Repeat daily if there is cold or congestion in the nose or sinus trouble.

(iii) BENEFITS: Cleanses and disinfects nasal passage; respiration becomes easy; cools the brain and calms the nervous system.

(iv) SPECIAL INSTRUCTIONS: Do not use tap water without boiling the same and adding salt.

Use warm water, if there is congestion in the nose. Do the practice before your regular yoga practices. Never do the practice before going to sleep. Be relaxed during the practice and do not hurry while sucking the water through one nostril nor strain yourself. Do not take in too much quantity of water in the nose by a feeding cup, etc.

8.4 KAPAL BHATI (*Exercise for the Sinuses*)

The process is of oxygenation vigorously through nostrils.

(i) METHOD: Stand in relaxed position, arms on sides. Exhale completely and concentrate on neck and face. Start quick inhalation and exhalation vigorously through both the nostrils (take a small quantity of breath and at once throw it out). Do this in one continuous cycle of rounds in quick succession, keeping your face and neck muscles relaxed. After each cycle of rounds, take a deep breath. Use kerchief to clean the mucus if there is any. Inhalation and exhalation should be even; maintain the same speed without pause. Do four or six cycles or rounds but if you feel giddy do not repeat it.

(ii) BENEFITS: Exercise for the sinuses; cleanses the upper respiratory passage by removing mucus and providing massage to the membrane; facial and neck muscles get activated.

9

UNDERSTANDING OF PRANAYAMA

9.1 INTRODUCTION

Pranayama is the fourth step in the systematic study of Yoga. Its full significance has to be properly understood and appreciated. It consists of two components, PRAN + AYAMA: PRANA is translated by Shri Yogendraji as bioenergy and AYAMA means control or discipline. The real meaning of Pranayama, therefore, is control of bioenergy. Prana is an essential living activity-agent that works in the human body and makes the various functions of the body possible.

There are five principal PRANAS and five other (secondary) pranas, including one overall (Mukhyaprana); they flow along well-marked channels and each has specific functions to perform, associated with physiological organs. The five major Pranas with their functions are:

PRANA : Breathing associated with respiratory system giving vitality to the human system. It helps the movement of prana upwards.

APANA : Active below the navel and moves downwards. It governs elimination — function of the kidneys, bladder, colon, rectum and reproductive organs.

SAMANA : It governs assimilation and digestion of food and other metabolic processes.

UDANA : Energy used in sensory perception and brain are activated by this prana.

VYANA : To maintain circulation of blood throughout the body.

The stoppage of pulse and heart, indifference to heat and cold, the act of burying alive underground, immunity to the effects of chemicals are a afew of the powers that can be achieved by the mastery or control over prana. The yogis mobilise this energy and will it to any desired part of the body to cause healing. Prana is not vayu or breath but the vital force or life-force which expresses itself in different ways at different levels of consciousness. But since outside air is surcharged with a maximum percentage of prana, all importance is given to the yogic method of deep breathing. One can absorb larger quantities of atmospheric energy this way. But how can one do this unless one has learnt to expand the lungs to one's fullest capacity from the apex to the base. Very few people know the correct method and importance of correct breathing.

It is also known that the yogis consciously control the breathing rate and bring their normal rate to 8 or 10 times a minute instead of the average rate of 14 to 16 times a minute. It is said that the span of one's life is determined by the number of breaths one breathes. This is amplified in the case of animals. Those animals whose rate of breathing is fast have a shorter span of life, for example:

Rabbit : rate of breathing 42/minute, lives for 10 years approximately.
Horse : rate of breathing 35/minute, lives for 20 to 30 years.
Elephant : rate of breathing 5/minute, lives for 150 to 200 years.
Tortoise : rate of breathing 3/minute, lives for 300 to 400 years.

This means dissipated breathing brings early death, while regulation, control and fewer times you breathe prolong life.

9.2 RESPIRATORY SYSTEM AND ITS CARE

Respiration is concerned not only with the breathing and lung structure but also with the bloodstream since oxygen is supplied to the blood via the respiratory system. The air enters from the nostrils and passes through the larynx into the Trachea (windpipe) which divides it into two branches (bronchi), one to each lung. Each bronchus gives rise to smaller branches and breaks up into bronchioles and finally terminates in the tiny air cells of the lungs called alveoli. It is in the alveoli that interchange of gases take place between air and blood. The blood absorbs oxygen and gives off the waste or carbon dioxide. Purified and oxygenated blood is returned to the left side of the heart by the pulmonary veins and then distributed to the whole body. In short, lungs are the factory where the refining process takes place. If lungs are not in a proper condition or there is some blockage in the respiratory passage or you have shallow breathing or faulty breathing using only the upper part of the lungs it affects the respiratory system which in turn effects the circulatory system.

For yogic complete breath, where the lungs are utilized in their full capacity it is important to train the three sets of respiratory muscles: (a) the Diaphragm, (b) the Intercostal muscles, and (c) the Clavicular muscles (muscles round the armpit and collar bone). When all these three respiratory muscles coordinate well, the bony cage of ribs opens up well and the diaphragm descends down and the chest cavity is enlarged allowing the lungs to take in oxygen to its full capacity and the objective of complete breath is achieved. All this respiratory development is needed for hyper-oxygenation, keeping the brain function with clear blood and also keeping what is called reserve of oxygen. This is a good investment against disease like pleurisy, pneumonia, T.B. and other respiratory troubles. Remember, blood with low oxygen content is open to disease.

"PRANA and CHITTA are two sides of the same coin." Breathing again is correlated to your mental and emotional life. When you are angry, your breathing is fast, jerky, uneven and short and when you are calm and tranquil, watch your breath and you will find it smooth, even and rhythmic. Breathing indicates emotional instability or mental agitation or disturbance specially through rhythm. Yogis use breathing as a means of controlling Prana and Chitta. Harmonious and rhythmic breathing quietens the mind and brings about mental equilibrium — your anxiety and tension is dissolved. Your power of concentration improves with much less disturbance and distractions.

Prana is supplied by food, air and solar energy. It is manifested in different forms — when it flows in the nerves it is called nervous energy; in the muscles it is muscular energy; in the seminal fluid it is sexual energy. In its finer form it becomes mental power, thought power, power of imagination etc. Hence, energies of the vital life force are discharged through nervous system containing 72,000 nerves or nadis through Prana Vahaka or nerve impulses. Raja Yoga reminds us that the mind-body has only one life force. Prana also is a cosmic phenomenon. The ancient yogis definitely thought about it, not only as a physical reality but also that it covers a universal aspect of world energy principle, prevading and sustaining life.

9.3 A WORD OF CAUTION

It is dangerous to dabble in traditional pranayama without proper preparation and guidance of an expert teacher. It demands a well-regulated life in yogic discipline and purity where the mind is purged of base desires and tendencies, otherwise one may ruin one's nerves and brain and even incur risk of insanity.

A SIMPLE SYSTEM of preliminary pranayamas has been evolved by Shri Yogendraji whereby the respiratory mechanism is fully harmonised and organically developed which also leads to regulation and control of respiratory movement. All this is very easy, safe and useful to the modern man. Yogendra Pranayama No. 1 is a conditioning process to establish harmony at the respiratory level. Nos. 2,3 and 4 are specific methods of breathing to give exercise to a particular set of respiratory muscles. In course of time, you will be able to coordinate all the respiratory muscles for a yogic complete breath. Breathing through alternate nostrils is also included to regulate the varied effects of breath on the body and mind.

9.4 PRANAYAMA PRACTICES CAN HELP IN MANY WAYS

1. To develop the respiratory organs and to improve your vital capacity (lungs capacity).
2. To aid the circulation of the blood.
3. To produce inner, organic and natural harmony.
4. To provide efficient control over the respiratory movements.
5. Longer and deeper breathing produces sedative effect on nerves.
6. Useful for emotional control.
7. Helps in steadiness of the mind and in concentration.
8. More bioenergy (Prana) is absorbed and stored in the body.
9. Preparation for meditation takes place when breathing becomes subtle.

9.5 GENERAL PRECAUTIONS

1. Breathe in and breathe out through the nose only.
2. Do it without producing any sound.
3. Relax your body and keep your mind calm before commencing pranayama. Do it as indicated in the guide table or after Savasana.
4. Keep timing by counting numbers mentally. Equalize your breathing in and breathing out.

5. Do it morning and evening - twice a day is sufficient. To progress, add one count every week to reach to a maximum of 8 or 10 seconds in each inhalation/exhalation.
6. Take a few normal breaths after one type of pranayama and generally start with slow exhalation.
7. Practise not more than three types of pranayamas in one sitting and do not exceed the total of thirty rounds — ten rounds in each pranayama.
8. Concentrate on your breathing. It is very important to do it smoothly, gently without strain. Try to acquire a steady control over your respiratory movements. It should be one uniform, continuous steady movement both in inhalation and exhalation, without the pause of retention or suspension.

9.6 INSTITUTIONAL YOGENDRA PRANAYAMAS

9.6.1 Yogendra Panayama No. 1 *(In Standing Position)*

(i) FOR CONDITIONING PROCESS: A simple form of Ujjayi.
To put your attention on the normal flow of breathing.
To give a feeling of ease in practice.
To make you time-conscious.
To acquire a gentle control over the respiratory movement and gradually to prolong the act of respiration.

(ii) METHOD

1. Stand erect in a relaxed manner with feet apart.
2. Inhale slowly, comfortably and smoothly in a continuous manner for, say, 4 seconds.
3. At the end of inhalation, start exhaling with the same speed of inhalation — 4 seconds i.e., equalize inhalation and exhalation timings.
4. Let there be no jerks or strain. Do it effortlessly and concentrate on the uninterrupted flow of breath.

(iii) FREQUENCY: Repeat 10 rounds starting with your easy count which you should be able to maintain. Gradually increase by one count every week and come to a count of 10 seconds.

Note: Keep timing either by looking at the watch or mentally counting "one-thousand-one", "one-thousand-two" etc. or counting numbers mentally at the same speed. Later, this practice can be done sitting, in a meditative posture.

(iv) BENEFITS: better oxygenation; even use of inspiratory and expiratory effort; sense of harmony; improved concentration.

YOGENDRA PRANAYAMA NO. 2
(INTERCOSTAL BREATHING)

9.6.2 Yogendra Pranayama No. 2 *(In Standing Position)*

Intercostal breathing or Rib breathing

(i) METHOD

1. Assume standing position as in Pranayama No. 1.
2. Place your hands on the lower portion of the ribs on either side as shown in Fig. 36a.

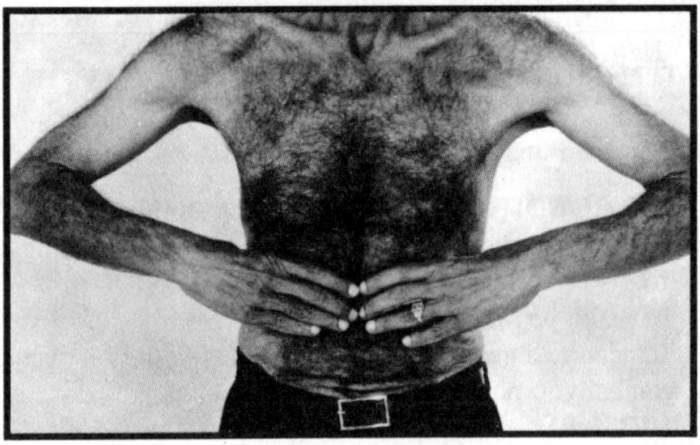

3. Now inhale in such a way that the lateral movement of the ribs is distinctly felt (Fig. 36b), by expanding the intercos-

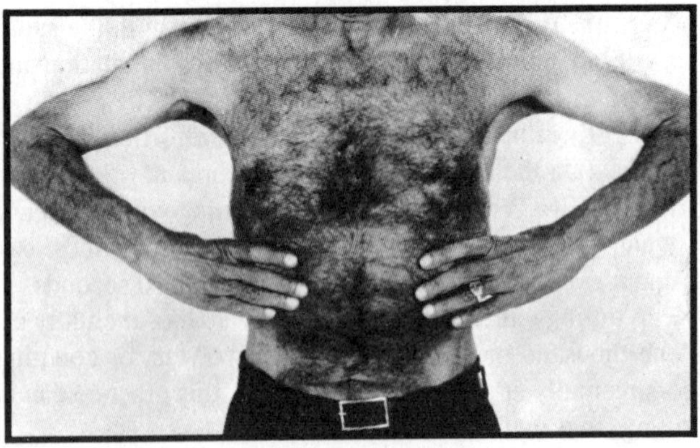

tal muscles — muscles in between the ribs (Fig. 36c). Do it to a count of five to manage easily.

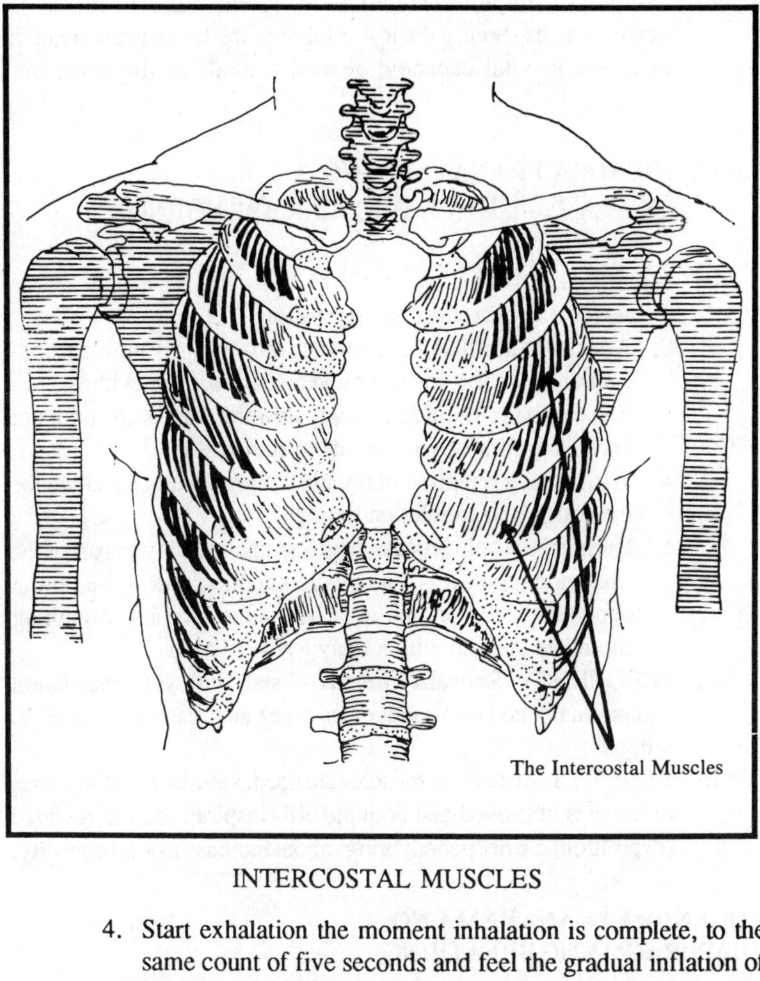

INTERCOSTAL MUSCLES

4. Start exhalation the moment inhalation is complete, to the same count of five seconds and feel the gradual inflation of the ribs — the lateral movement of the ribs is distinctly felt.
5. See that the abdomen is held in normal contour and there is no vertical movement of the boney cage.
6. Note that in every round you equalize your inhalation and exhalation to a count of five.

(ii) FREQUENCY: Repeat up to 10 rounds. Gradually add one count every week after starting with five initially.

Note: Do not attempt to increase the counts or the rounds beyond ten.

(iii) BENEFITS: Improves control of intercostal muscles; increases ventilation, especially the lower lobes of the lungs get activated; increases in vital capacity; general contour of the chest improves.

9.6.3 YOGENDRA PRANAYAMA NO. 3

(In Standing Position) (CLAVICULAR BREATHING)

(i) METHOD

1. Assume a relaxed standing position.
2. After normal exhalation, begin to inhale gently upward, concentrating on the vertical movement of the upper chest.
3. Raise also the shoulders slowly upwards and keep count not exceeding four or six seconds to start with.
4. Without any retention of breath, slowly exhale. Equalize the inhalation and exhalation timings.
5. During the whole process keep abdomen and lower part of the ribs under control — the whole attention should be on the upper chest region and area below the armpits. Breathing should be smooth without any jerks or strain.

(ii) FREQUENCY: Repeat 10 rounds — start with your easy count and gradually add one count every week and reach a count of 10 seconds.

(iii) BENEFITS: Accessory muscles are used; ventilation of the apex of lungs is improved and both *puraka* (inspiration) and *rechaka* (expiration) are deepened; brings about increase in vital capacity.

YOGENDRA PRANAYAMA NO. 4
(DIAPHRAGMATIC BREATHING)

(i) METHOD

1. Lie supine and bend legs at knees, keeping the soles of the feet on the ground.
2. Place one hand on abdomen, the other hand on the side. Relax the abdomen.
3. With inhalation, allow abdomen to rise up, but not too much.

DIAPHRAGM: An important muscle in breathing separating the abdomen from the thoracic cavity.

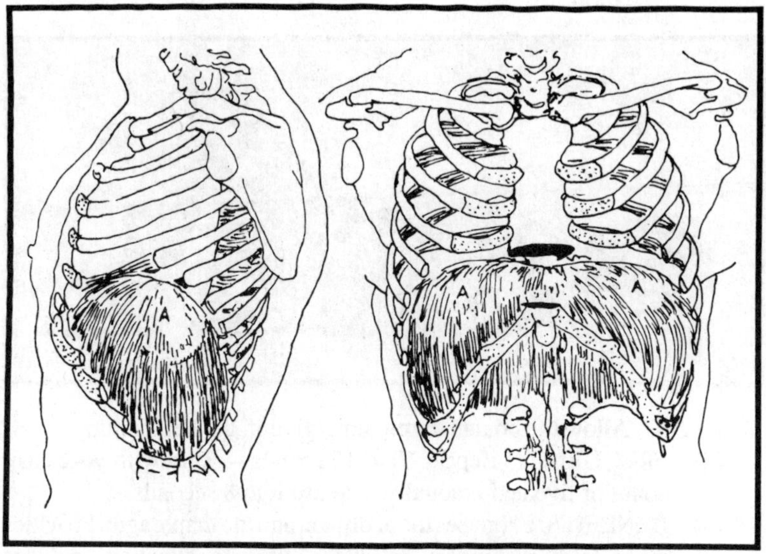

Fig. 37a The Diaphragm A-Tendon

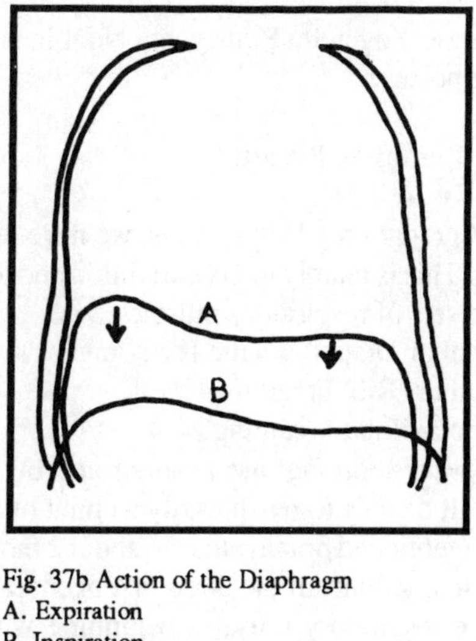

Fig. 37b Action of the Diaphragm
A. Expiration
B. Inspiration

With inspiration it contracts, flattening out downward and with expiration it is restored to its relaxed domeshape position.

4. With exhalation, allow abdomen to descend (Fig. 37c).
5. Keep count and equalise the timing for inhalation and exhalation.

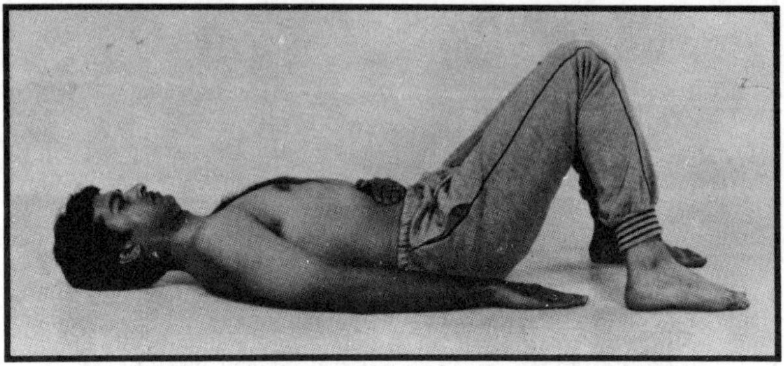

6. Allow the counts to remain at five in the beginning.

(ii) FREQUENCY: Repeat 10 to 15 rounds — start with your easy count of five and gradually increase it to 8 seconds.

(iii) BENEFITS: Exercises the abdomen and the diaphragm. Provides relief from respiratory troubles; cures constipation; reduces obesity; aids relaxation.

Note: Later, practise Yogendra Pranayama No.4 in sitting position in a meditative posture.

9.6.5 The Yogic Complete Breath

As a process of preparatory Pranayamas, we have learnt three distinct types of breathing. This is mainly to give attention and to provide exercise separately to three sets of respiratory muscles, viz.

1) Abdominal or Diaphragmatic breathing — Y.P. No. 4
2) Intercostal or 'Rib' breathing — Y.P. No. 2
3) Upper or clavilular breathing — Y.P. No. 3

By practising every morning and evening and by adding one count every week you will be able to reach easily a count of 8 or 10 seconds in each of the above-mentioned pranayamas in about 2 months time. You are now in a position to combine all the three in Yogendra Pranayama No. 1 and involve all the respiratory muscles beginning with the diaphragm, intercostal and clavicular, without any exaggerated movements. By doing this, the entire repiratory organism and the three distinct parts of the lungs

— Superior, Middle and Inferior lobes get thoroughly ventilated as the chest cavity is expanded in all directions as shown by arrows in Fig. 38.

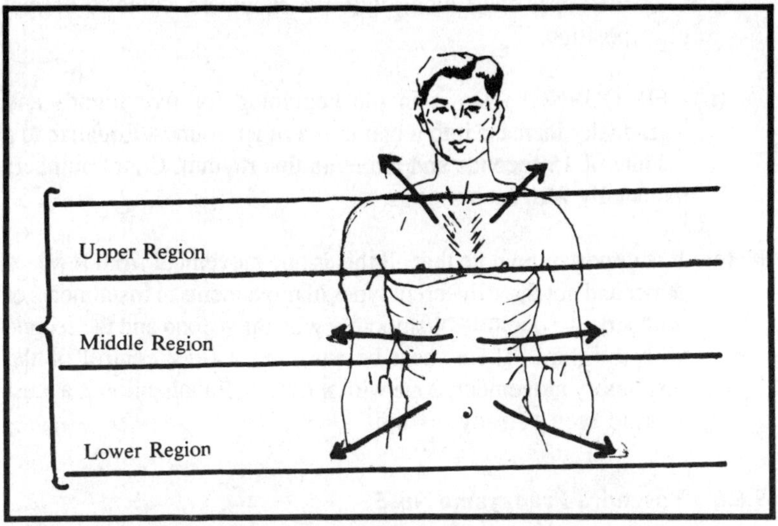

The Yogic Complete Breath from three levels or Regions.

The most important is Intercostal Diaphragmatic breathing (Y.P. No. 4 + Y.P. No. 2) and add to this a little, upper part (clavicular breathing).

(i) METHOD

1. Sit in any meditative posture (Sukhasana/Vajrasana).

BREATHING IN

2. First breathe in from lower region through diaphragmatic breathing, pushing the front wall of the abdomen a little, to a count of five (diaphragm pushed down).
3. Then expand the lower part of the ribs (middle region) outwards and forwards by intercostal breathing to a count of five or to your comfortable capacity (the rib-cage expanded). Fig. 38.
4. Finally add another count of five through clavicular breathing (upper region) by raising slowly the collar bones, shoulders and lifting the bony cage vertically. This will fill the upper portion of the chest (Apical portion of the lungs).

BREATHING OUT

5. Holding the chest, exhale first by withdrawing the abdomen in, then relax the expanded portion of lower ribs and finally the upper chest along with the shoulders, come to normal position.

(ii) FREQUENCY: Do it in the beginning for five rounds and gradually increase it to a maximum of ten rounds. Equalize to a count of 15 seconds and maintain this rhythm. Count numbers mentally with each round.

Note: It is important to note that all this is one movement from lower to upper and not three different types of movements in instalments or with jerks — one mixed smoothly with the second and the second with the third. There must be ease and a finer control of the respiratory movement, done without strain. Equalization is a must so as to keep a steady rhythm.

9.6.6 Yogendra Pranayama No. 5
(Sunyaka or *Vacuum Breathing)*

(i) METHOD

1. Sit in Sukhasana or Vajrasana or Padmasana.
2. Breathe in and out normally a few times. When short inhalation is complete slowly begin throwing out the breath in one long continuous manner drawing the abdomen inwards towards the spine till you feel that you cannot exhale any more.
3. When exhalation is complete, suspend breathing, i.e., do not either inhale or exhale and be absolutely still. The abdomen looks like a deep valley (Fig. 39). Suspension of breath occurs and eyes are fixed on a point or focussed on the tip of the nose simultaneously.
4. Keep this up for five seconds to begin with, gradually increasing it to thirty seconds.
5. Now relax the diaphragm and inhale slowly without any strain. Then exhale slowly till your normal rhythm is maintained.

(ii) FREQUENCY: Practise this for ten rounds, taking a pause of a few seconds in between (normal rounds of breathing) and then start the next round.

(iii) BENEFITS: Effective in case of weak stomach and sluggish colon; generally creates hunger and feeling of increased vigour; aids circulation and purification of the blood through internal pressure upon the abdominal viscera.

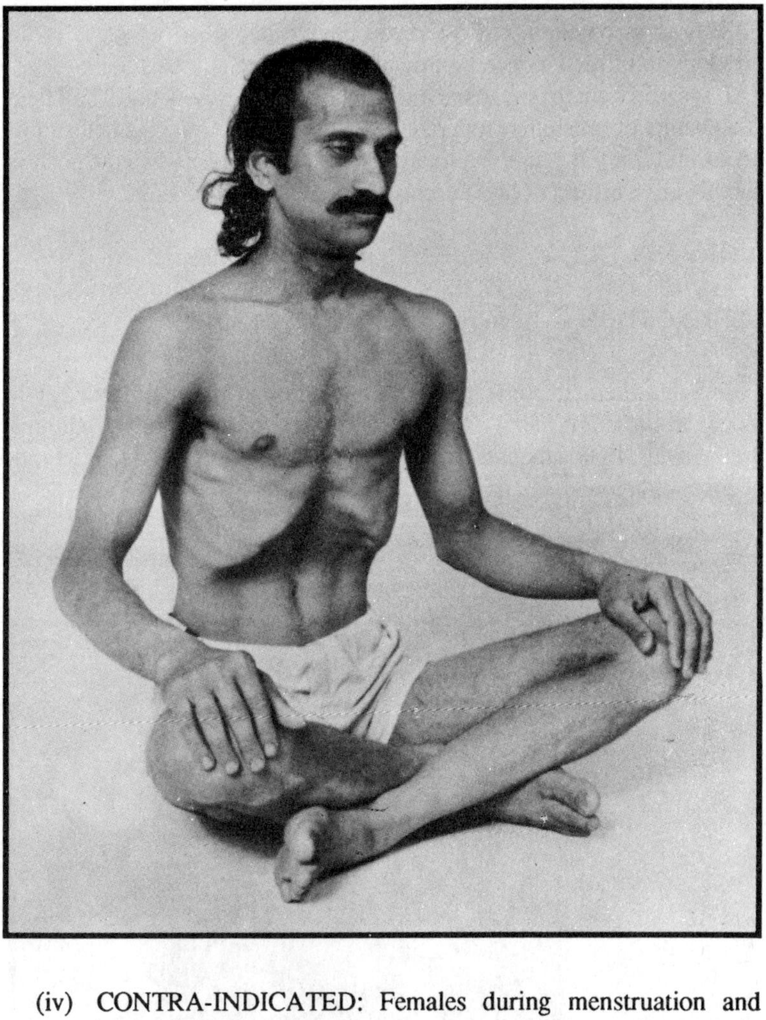

(iv) CONTRA-INDICATED: Females during menstruation and pregnancy and also those with weak heart and lungs should avoid this method.

A TRADITIONAL PRANAYAMA

9.6.7 Yoga Alternate Breathing*

(Suryabhedana or Anuloma-viloma Pranayama)

*Regulate the flow of positive and negative energy by Yoga Alternate Breathing

This is to be attempted after you have made good progress in the previous simplified Yogendra Pranayamas covered in 9.6.1.

It is significant to note that in human beings every hour and a half there is a change of breathing from one nostril to another (one becomes more active and free). It Nature's process to keep balance between the positive and negative effects of breath on both the body and the mind.

RIGHT NOSTRIL	— Positive (HOT)	— Solar Influences (Surya)
LEFT NOSTRIL	— Negative (COLD)	— Lunar influence (Chandra)

In Yoga alternate use of the right and left nostril is recommended at the Yoga Institute of Santa Cruz Bombay out of the many traditional pranayamas. In this there is a measured breathing according to a set ratio between inhalation, retention and exhalation.

(i) METHOD

1. Assume a meditative posture and use thumb and last two fingers or little finger alone for breathing.

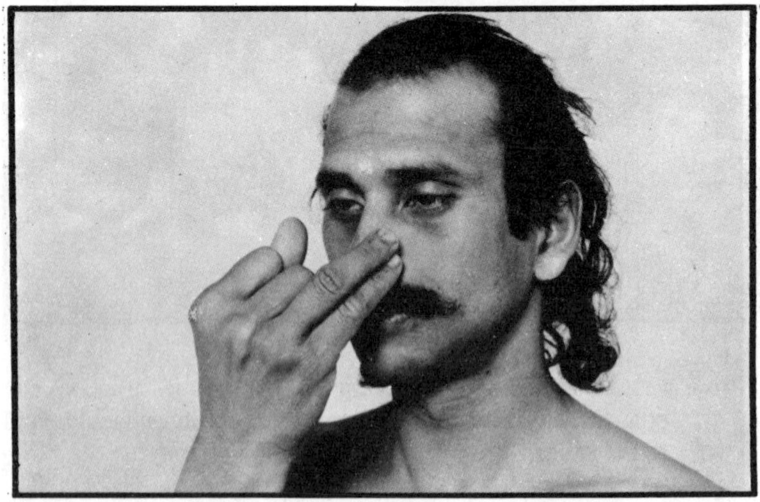

2. Have 2 seconds (1) *suspension* or pause before undertaking deep breathing.
3. Breathe in slowly and uniformly through the right nostril to a count of 2 seconds (2) *inhalation* closing your left nostril with the last two fingers of the right hand.
4. Hold the breath, by immediately closing the right nostril with the thumb, to a count of 4 seconds (3) *retention*—both nostrils closed.
5. Breathe out gently through the left nostril closing the right one with the thumb to a count of 2 seconds (4) *exhalation*.
6. Breathe in immediately through the left nostril to a count of 2 seconds (5) *inhalation* keeping the right nostril closed.
7. Retention of breath as before, closing both the nostrils, to a count of 4 seconds (6) *retention*.
8. Breathe out through the right nostril by closing the left one for 2 seconds (7) *exhalation*.
9. A period of expiratory standstill or a pause natural to a complete round for 2 seconds (8) *suspension*.

(ii) FREQUENCY: 4 rounds. Practise both in the morning and in the evening.

(iii) INITIAL RHYTHM: (Time to be regulated)
— 2:2:4:2:2:4:2:2 = 3 breaths/minute

(iv) LATER ON (Adjust to)
— 3:3:6:3:3:6:3:3 = 2 breaths/minute

(v) FINALLY (maximum) (Adjust to)
— 4:4:8:4:4:8:4:4 = 1 breath/minute

(vi) BENEFITS: It improves digestion; brings regulation and unification of breathing movement; brings harmony between all acts of respiration; provides beneficial effects on heart and brain.

* Based on Shri Yogendraji — Journal of the Yoga Institute, Vol. XXVIX – Oct 1983. No. 3.

10

THE 3-R's: REST, RECREATION AND RELAXATION

10.1 INTRODUCTION

The Modern Complexities of life, with its stress and strain, have made living a constant source of conflict and tension. In a big city with its usual busy life accompanied by hurry and worry and a constant struggle for existence, the common man, many a time, feels tired and exhausted. Tension seems to cripple him and he finds himself unable to cope with his day-to-day work. It is common sense that the body and mind which are in constant activity, need some sort of relaxation, as a stop-gap process. But unfortunately this art of relaxation is not known to many. People are agitated, temperamental, sentimental and emotional. People who have greater responsibilities and ambitions lead a life which is even more active. It is this type of condition that causes more harm and has an evident effect on both body and mind.

10.2 REST IS THE PRINCIPLE OF RELAXATION

In any case, it becomes necessary that you break the period of activity by *rest*. The wear and tear of the body is compensated during sleep by Nature. This helps in maintaining the steady rhythm of life. It is in this way that the efficiency is maintained at the level of the body and the mind. But many people do not sleep till midnight, or their sleep is disturbed by dreams or external environmental factors. Sometimes it may be some worry that keeps them awake till late at night. They perhaps resort to sleeping pills which are used widely in the West. This is because natural sleep does not come to them. The chemicals contained in these sleeping pills (tranquillizers) are harmful for the brain and they can do damage to an extent that cannot be foretold. *Remember, what is needed more than sleep is rest.*

10.3 QUIET ENTERTAINMENT MAKES FOR REAL RELAXATION

The recreating process means to recreate the body and mind because something was lost, and to keep the balance one has to gain that back. This recreation can be more physical and less mental or vice versa. Football, for example, is a heavy game, you may be enjoying it but you are using more energy. Similarly, playing chess seriously may involve much mental preoccupation. You must understand that leisurely *quiet* entertainment relaxes you where there is no spirit of competition or show. Swimming is a very recreative process. A walk through a park; a small climb on a little hillock; a trip to the beach or anything wherein you seek a change of scene and activity are all well worth planning. The housewife in the middle of her never-ending chores equally needs such short breaks at intervals. Spending time in gardening has both physical and mental aspects of recreation. One must, however, avoid entertainment which leads to *excitement* and results in *exhaustion*.

10.4 TOO MUCH ACTIVITY AND NO ACTIVITY — BOTH ARE HARMFUL

There is an example of a man who is greedy and who cares a lot for money. He is ambitious and has too many needs and wants. He is a paid slave during the working day and even thereafter. He forgets that it is necessary to have a period of rest. In some countries like Canada and Russia, in many factories, they provide break periods and call them Yoga breaks. In that period, workers do some movement, breathing exercises and enjoy relaxation. They found that this recreating process increased their efficiency up to 17 per cent and the person was able to do more work. Remember that even in the case of a horse-driven carriage, the horse may collapse if given no food and no rest.

There is another class of people who have nothing to do—a leisurely drive in the evening or going to the club and coming back again. They suffer because of inactivity - a disease of laziness where the machine is not used at all. These people being of a highly sentimental and emotional constitution are not able to sleep at night and complain of all kinds of symptoms. They fail to realise that rest is necessary only when they feel the beginning of fatigue.

10.5 THE BASIC PROBLEM IS ONE OF TENSION

Everything seems to be geared to *tension*. We work under tension, eat under tension, love under tension and we even rest under tension! Tension seems to be the root cause of ill-health - physical and mental. The nerves cannot relax because of their fixed grip on the muscles and the muscles cannot relax because the nerves are tense. In purely physical tension, there is a constriction of muscles whether at work or at play; restriction in joint flexibility and in breathing; poor circulation, pain, irritability. This may result in hyper-activity of organs bringing about some physio-chemical changes in the physiological system. But in our present-day keyed-up existence, there is a constant *nervous tension* originating from the mind and expressed through our nervous system. The mind having a vicious hold on the body does not allow muscular and bodily relaxation. It may be mental agitation and conflict, anxiety and worry or you may be pushed around due to lack of emotional stability.

Tension can be divided into two categories - neuro-muscular and mental, either of which becomes an oppressive barrier in the art of relaxation.

10.6 RELAXATION, CENTRAL IDEA IN MODERN YOGA

Relaxation is, therefore rightly a central idea in modern yoga. It tries to break down all unnecessary physical *tensions*, tries to maintain harmony in the body-mind relationship and, above all, provides mental poise and serenity.

10.6.1 Yogic Asanas

The yoga method of doing various cultural *asanas* with its emphasis on the stretch part of muscles rather than the contraction of the active muscles, its important contributive salient feature of coordination between the muscular and the respiratory systems giving a pause period of respiratory standstill, re-educates, your muscular movements, contributes towards suppleness, poise and control of body and mind. All this leads to complete physical repose-the mind is made free from any kind of physical anxiety.

10.6.2 Yogic Breathing Method

The deep breathing process where the respiratory act is harmonized and controlled, brings about mental equilibrium and considerable relaxation which have a soothing effect on the nerves.

10.6.3 Special Psychosomatic Practices

But our mind needs much more attention. The mind is in a constant flux of thoughts, feelings and sensations and most of the trouble in this modern age is mental and emotional because of heightened *nervous strain*. We call the more relaxing practices in our course, *psychosomatic* practices. These are the best type of practices which have a direct impact on the mind, thinking, feelings, and emotions and bring about ultimately, the desired psycho-physical changes.

These practices will bring about a state of neuro-muscular relaxation with an increase in energy content of the body, in the shortest possible time. They relieve us of psychosomatic disturbances. They give us a feeling of freshness, provide energy, physical rest and mental poise. They help us to achieve steadiness of mind, unifying our experience and harmonizing us with a higher state of consciousness.

10.7 SOME IMPORTANT TIPS

A heavy dinner at night is not advisable. Due to digestion trouble, gases and gurgling, sleep is disturbed. Take food one hour before going to bed. No burden on memory should be carried before retiring like reading an exciting novel or entertaining romantic ideas. The mind and body should be kept free as far as possible from any pressure - social, economical, environmental, emotional, political, etc. If one works when already tired, one uses three times the usual amount of energy - the damage is greater than imagined generally. Standing is more tiring than walking.

Dodging a job gives you double fatigue. Do not depend upon tranquillizers, analgesics or laxatives. How well one rests means more than how long one sleeps. Relaxed rest is effective in restoring energy. Never get impatient about your progress towards perfect relaxation. Go forward steadily and persistently and never lose faith in yourself.

10.8 SPECIAL PSYCHOSOMATIC PRACTICES

"Relaxation quickly recuperates, regalvanises the nerve centres, collects the scattered forces, reinvigorates the whole body."

- Shri Yogendraji

If these psychosomatic practices are learned properly and if right time is devoted to these practices (not less than 10 minutes at the minimum) daily, one will have found a new freedom from everyday worry and tension. One is then able to release one's nervous *tension* and has learnt the art of leading a *carefree* life.

10.8.1 Yogendra Nispanda Bhava

With learning to condition the mind through meditative postures described in the beginning of the course, you may have achieved some progress. The number of thoughts and their intensity must have been considerably reduced if you have sufficiently practised. This brings down the nervous agitation and *quietens* the mind.

However, in Yogendra Nispanda Bhava you have to make use of the sense of hearing (mechanics of sound) and, through it, achieve still greater *quietness* of mind - an unmoved condition which no disturbance can affect. Sit in a relaxed position, reclining against the wall, listen to a sound of low intensity, a rhythmic sound or a sound of a fading-out nature (like the sound of a passing by car or aeroplane). This listening is to be done in a *passive manner*. This passivity, when it deepens, leads to a deeper *quietness* where the hold of the mind on the body is loosened and it withdraws, narrowing the beam of consciousness.

Yogendra Nispanda Bhava (Motionless State of Mind)

Nis	: Negative
Panda	: Movement
Bhava	: State of mind.

(i) METHOD: Sit relaxed reclining against the wall.. Properly adjust your legs, feet, arms and hands to a comfortable position (Fig.41). Sit motionless and feel quiet. Keep attention on sound

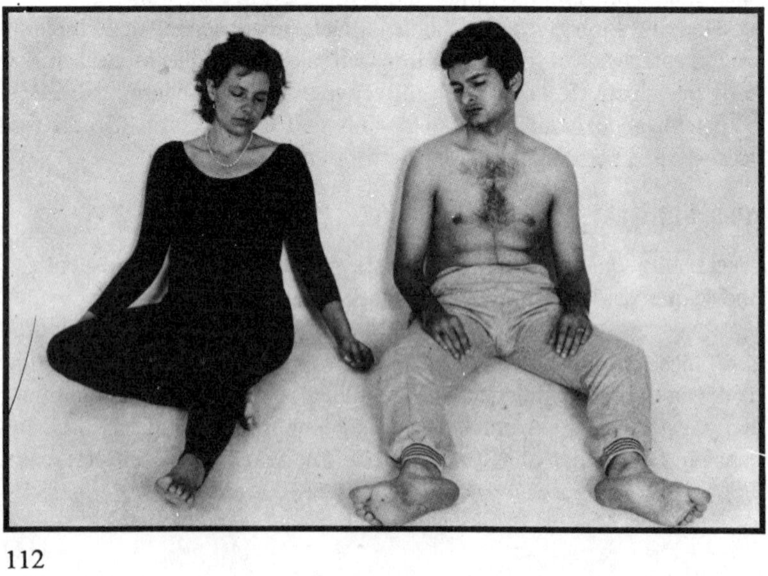

— preferably a low-intensity or a fading sound or a rhythmic sound, for example, of a time-piece. Cultivate the passive attitude of listening. Remain passive and get completely absorbed in the sound.

(ii) RHYTHM: Normal breathing.

(iii) DURATION: 10 to 15 minutes.

(iv) BENEFITS: Introspective training of mind. Release of tension. Feeling of being physically and mentally relaxed. Subjective experience of quietude. Ideal technique for cultivating passivity.

Note: One can do it sitting on a chair or sofa in the office or at home (Fig. 42).

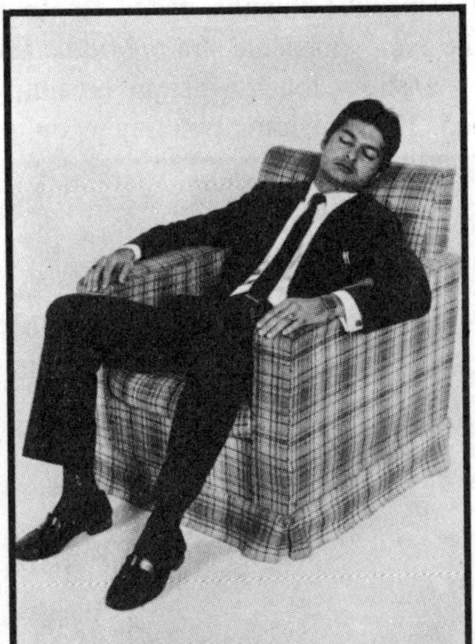

10.8.2 Yoni Mudra

The main purpose of this practice is to withdraw the mind from sense objects and take you in a mechanical way to the stage of abstraction (Pratyahara). This is the best way to give rest to your turbulent mind in a conscious way and to conserve energy. The stoppage of outward tendency itself directly brings about a change in the state of mind and feeling. Sitting in a meditative posture, holding the arms in a particular way with thumb and fingers tackling various senses (hearing,smell and taste), it combines a sort of neuro-muscular training and an exercise for endurance. Giving pressure on the ears by pressing the lobes through the respective thumbs gives a vibrating sound from the brain and helps in localising the mind or maybe you hear the inner sound of your breathing as you inhale and exhale. Synchronise your mind with it. Yoni Mudra is much praised and is highly recommended for higher practices in Yoga. It is rightly termed Yoni Mudra, because with its aid, the yoga aspirant can reach, through subjective approach, after avoiding all objective contacts, his true origin or Yoni which this practice symbolises.

Yoni Mudra (*Symbol of True Origin*)

(i) METHOD:Sitting in a meditative posture, preferably Padmasana, close various organs (senses). Close ears, pressing the lobes with the respective thumbs. Index finger on eyelashes after closing the eyes - no undue strain. Middle fingers on either side of nose - a slight touch wherein breathing could be easily maintained. The remaining two fingers on the upper and lower

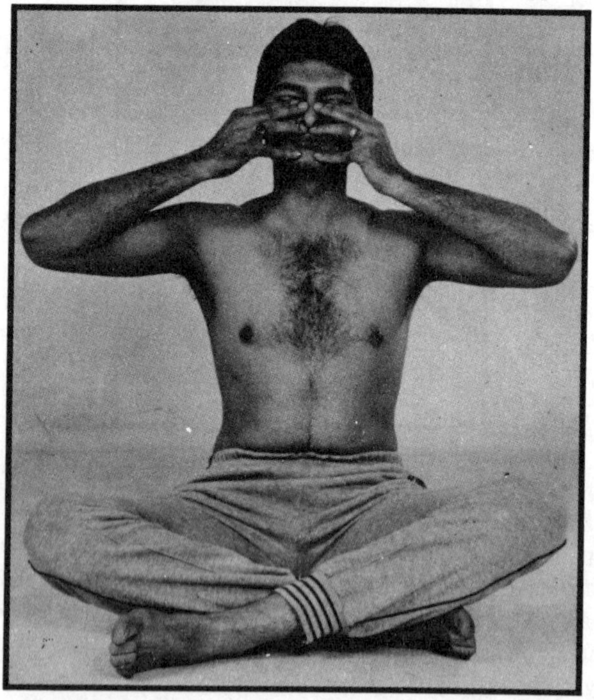

lips (Fig. 43). Retain the pose - keep yourself motionless as far as possible. The mind is to be given no work. If you can hear the breathing sound, put your mind in listening to it or vibrating sound at the ears.

(ii) RHYTHM: Normal breathing.

(iii) DURATION: 10 to 15 minutes.

(iv) BENEFITS: Gives rest to a turbulent mind; conserves energy; controls external senses; leads to pratyahara (abstraction); induces joy of solitude.

10.8.3 Savasana

The technique consists in lying supine, motionless, like a corpse, with arms and legs extended to their full length and to offer no resistance against the pull of gravity by working on the principle of 'Let go'. This partial relaxation should be done in sections attending to different limbs and joints until they all become deeply relaxed, limp and heavy. There is a process of relaxation from partial to general and deep relaxation. In deep relaxation, the metabolic rate goes from a minimum of 10 to a maximum of 20 per cent which has an added advantage which the ancient yogis knew all about.

"True relaxation would mean a complete resignation of the body to the laws of gravity, the mind to nature and the entire energy transferred to a deep dynamic breathing." —Shri Yogendraji

In the advanced stage, systematically relax and inhibit afferent and efferent (sensory and motor) nervous impulses. The process is to withdraw attention consciously in stages from the sixteen vital zones (listed in subsequent pages) starting from the feet and slowly working up to the head, leading to a deep state of relaxation which may culminate in Yoga Nidra - the dreamless sleep of the yogis. The whole body can switch off, as it were. This especially restores and recoups energy and re-invigorates the whole body in the minimum of time.

In a desert oasis, people lie on the stomach like Makarasana for 15-20 minutes and look fresh and regain energy.

Savasana *(A Corpse Posture)*
(First and Second Stages of Partial Relaxation)

(i) METHOD: Lie down supine. Maintain 20" distance between feet, hands 10" to 12" apart (Fig. 44). Relax all parts - allow body to "Let go" to gravity. Keep your attention on different parts of the body one after the other and feel if these are relaxed. Break up tension from legs, feet, arms, hands, palms; check that the shoulders are flat; head and neck carefully adjusted. With each exhalation, feeling of sinking-down and still down, let go resistance against the pull of gravity.

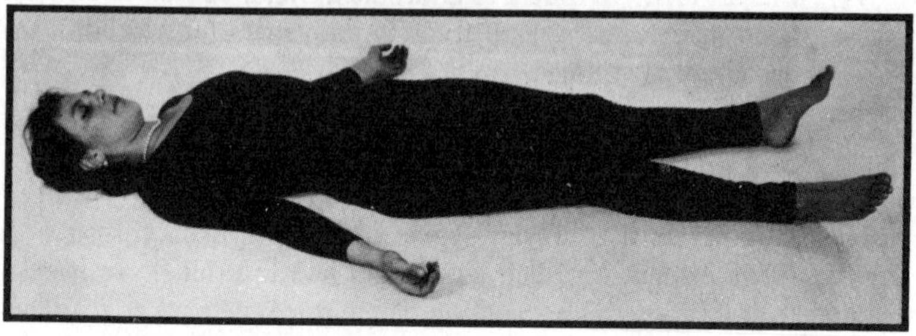

(ii) RHYTHM: Normal breathing.

(iii) FREQUENCY : 8 to 10 minutes.

(iv) BENEFITS : Provides complete rest and muscular relaxation. Transfers energy from overused parts to other vital organs; helps in psychosomatic disorders; induces better sleep.

Third Stage of General Relaxation

(i) METHOD: After doing the first two stages, working on the principle of 'Let go', and breaking up of tension to relax particular parts, in this third stage conscious attention is withdrawn by stages from the sixteen vital zones of the body from the toes to the top of the skull - on each zone stay for 30 seconds approximately - visualize the part, its shape, size, texture, colour, etc., and then withdraw the impulse and take it to the next part till you finish all the zones in this particular sequence. Repeat the cycle for any residual tension left over. Attend to normal rhythmic breathing. The zones are:

1. Toes
2. Ankles
3. Kness
4. Thighs (simultaneously with the arms)
5. Anus
6. Generative organ
7. Navel
8. Stomach

9. Heart
10. Neck
11. Lips
12. Tip of the nose
13. Eyes
14. Space between the eyebrows
15. Forehead
16. Top of the skull

(ii) DURATION : 8 to 10 minutes.

(iii) BENEFITS: Establishes muscular equilibrium and complete relaxation; renews strength and re-invigorates the whole body; good for building up heart tissues; pulse-rate and blood pressure go down; helps in psychosomatic disorders.

10.8.4 Makarasana (*The Crocodile Posture*)

Recommended for women for partial relaxation.

(i) METHOD: Lie down on the abdomen with the front of the body in contact with ground. Legs stretched at full length - partially separated. Arms folded and head resting thereon (Fig. 45). Work on the principle of 'Let Go' and offer no resistance against gravity

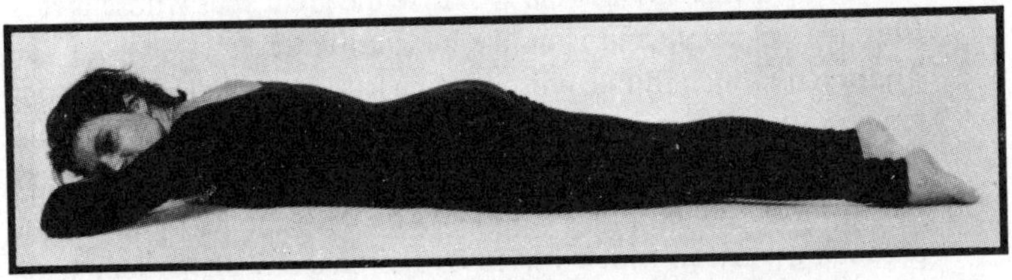

pull. Direct your attention to the lower parts of your body - the toes, the calves, thighs etc. and gradually move upwards to the head. Close the eyes and remain motionless. Put your mind to breathing and let the body consciousness fade away. Remain placid and motionless.

(ii) RHYTHM : Breathing slow, normal and rhythmic.

(iii) DURATION:10/15 minutes - practise it at mid-day or evening.

(iv) BENEFITS:Good posture for rest; good muscular relaxation; transfer of energy from over-used parts to other vital organs; helps in psychosomatic disorders; induces better sleep.

11

ALL ABOUT DIET IN A NUTSHELL

The food habits of a people depend on various factors such as geographical, historical, climatic and hereditary and these more or less determine the diet for most of us. However, it is wrong to be entirely governed by such factors. There should be a sense of discrimination and selection in what we eat in terms of good health and the kind of foods available.

11.1 WHY VEGETARIAN WAY OF LIFE?
Commonsense Point of View

1. Biological, anatomical and physiological evidence is in favour of man being a vegetarian. Man is akin to the great apes whose diet is fruit and vegetable and is unlike the carnivores.
2. The organs which filtrate poisons, such as kidneys and liver, are put to great strain by meat and eggs and can cause putrefaction in the digestive track.
3. Fat in meat (about 40%) is heavily of the saturated cholesterol producing variety which increases the chances of hardening of arteries and of heart diseases.
4. Meat is extra rich in proteins and is not easily digested. It contains urea and uric acid (a toxic compound). When it combines with the human blood, it gives rise to mental sickness, laziness and when it starts accumulating into some joints, it gives rise to joint pains, rheumatism and arthritis etc. Excessive protein can give rise to kidney stones.
5. Meat-eaters may also be troubled by poor elimination.
6. British and American statistics indicate that vegetarians are healthier, weigh less and their life-span is normally longer than their non-vegetarian counterparts. The Hunzas of Kashmir have a high longevity and enjoy freedom from disease since they are pure

vegetarians, living chiefly on whole grains, fresh fruits, vegetables, goat's milk and natural drinking water.

7. There is a great deal of truth in the saying that man becomes what he eats. The heavier the food, the grosser the body. Remember that your diet and your disposition are very closely related.
8. A well-balanced purely vegetarian SATTVIC DIET in Yoga is preferred to either a mixed or full flesh diet as
   a) it is easily digestible;
   b) by contrast it retains moisture and binds waste bulk for easy passage;
   c) it has less cholesterol;
   d) green and yellow leafy vegetables contain adequate vitamins which promote proper hormonal balance;
   e) it helps in relaxing the nerves;
   f) leafy vegetables are useful to preserve alkaline substance in the blood.

Note : It is a fallacy to believe that vegetarians do not get sufficient protein. Wheat combined with beans taken together is complete protein. Scientific studies clearly indicate that a starch-centred diet with the addition of fruits and vegetables supplies an excellent protein source. In skimmed milk when the fat is removed, the relative protein content doubles.

11.2 DIET-CLASSIFICATION

The diet can be divided into three types - one consisting entirely of meat another which is entirely vegetarian, and the third a mixture of the two. Yogis have given food a little higher value than merely its nutritive or chemical value. The characteristic Indian way of selecting a diet was by dividing it into three categories, depending upon the end-effects of the nutrients contained. *Rajasika* or a high-protein and energy-yielding diet is generally non-vegetarian. The *tamasika* or stale or bad food usually leads to malnutrition. Both these were, therefore, avoided by the yogis. They chose the *sattvika* kind of food made of pure energy-yielding constituents and completely vegetarian, because it is non-stimulating and the most ideal diet, especially for those engaged in higher mental pursuits and leading a quiet, sedentary life.

At present, scientists advise a fixed amount of calories, approximately 3,000 to be included in a person's daily diet. It has been lately discovered, however, that even 2,000 calories would be sufficient for certain classes of individuals. In fact, 3,000 calories could amount to over-eating which, in turn, might lead to diseases among the rich such as arthritis, diabetes, gout, etc.

Yoga believes that, first and foremost, one should know one's own body and its particular requirements. What may be lacking in one individual need not be lacking in another. Similarly, what can be assimilated by some may not be assimilated by others. For example, the diet for a man needing to put on weight cannot be the same as for one suffering from colitis. The same diet produces different reactions in different persons because of divergence in their individual digestive and assimilative capacities. Therefore, a fixed and standard diet with a specific number of calories is illogical, unscientific and, in fact, harmful to the body.

Yoga has prescribed its own balanced diet of pure, light and nutritious food. Four principles in the choice of food are: (1) Wholeness, (2) Freshness, (3) Alkalinity, and (4) Medicinal Value.

TYPES OF FOOD
According to Yoga

SATTVIC	RAJSIK	TAMSIK
Positive Non-irritant Foods	Negative Irritant Foods	Devitalizing Decomposed Foods Interia

1. SATTVIC: Pure, agreeable, nourishing and easily digestible.It urges purity of mind and inner strength and is conducive to higher thinking and pure intelligence, keeps the body in harmony, mind calm and gives you a cool temperament.

2. RAJSIK: Heavy protein, fats, difficult to digest and assimilate - the body has to waste energy. Excites emotions, causes disease, grief and pain and binds the soul through attachment to actions and their fruits.

3. TAMSIK: Stale and devitalising food. Processed and tinned foods. Also food reheated the next day. Leads to inertia and dullness and poisons the system.

According to Pandit Shiv Sharma, "The sattvic diet goes for the formation of the mind, i.e., the essence of food is for the mind and the rest of it for the body."

11.3 SELECTION OF FOODSTUFFS ACCORDING TO YOGIC DIET

Food Groups	**Foodstuffs**
Cereals	Wheat is preferable to rice, jowar, bajra, etc. Prepare chapatis made of whole-wheat grain. It is a good source of carbohydrates.
Milk	Milk is a complete food and so it must not beavoided. Dairy products such as butter, buttermilk, curds, cheese, ghee - all are recommended. It is valued for its protein, vitamin and mineral contents. For the vegetarian, it is the only source of animal or first-class proteins.
Pulses	Mung (green/black) dal is easy to digest and is therefore preferred to chana, tur, masur, etc. Beans also are a good source of protein, especially soyabean which has 43 per cent protein and a good amount of iron and vit. B Complex. Sprouted pulses are good sources of vitamin C.

Vegetables

Five most beneficial vegetables which are an excellent source of vitamins and minerals are:

(a) SPINACH	Provides iron, vitamins, calcium and for protein-building amino-acids. Other leafy vegetables like chowlai, methi (fenugreek), palak, mulla leaves and salad greens and raddish (muli) also contain minerals and vitamins.
(b) LADY'S FINGER (Bhendi)	Useful in all irritable states of intestines and for the genito-urinary organs.
(c) PARWAL (wild snake-gourd)	For vitality and vigour
(d) BRINJAL (Baigan)	Remedy for liver complaints.

(e) BITTER GOURD (Karela)		Excellent blood purifier. Good for gout, rheumatism and diseases of the spleen and liver. Medicinal doses of karela juice are recommended as a remedy in diabetes.

Roots and Tubers	Potatoes with jacket, suran (yam elephant), beetroot and carrots, are sources of carbohydrates. Carrot has Vitamin A, while potatoes have iron, magnesium, Vitamin B and C.
Sugar and Jaggery	Jaggery (gur) and honey are preferred to *white sugar*.* These are a good source of carbohydrates and concentrated source of energy.
Fruits	Citrus and other fruits are recommended except jack-fruit which has fibres and is difficult to digest. Avoid acidic, sour or unripe fruits. Fruits are a good source of vitamins.
Dry Fruits	Dates, figs, raisins, almonds, apricots, etc. are good sources of vitamins, if not treated chemically. They are also rich in carbohydrates and minerals.
*White Sugar	Dr Henry Schroeder, an eminent bio-chemist, is of the opinion that refining of raw sugar into white sugar removes 93 per cent of the ash which leads to chromium deficiency - one of the causes of the hardening of arteries and consequent heart diseases.
Oils and Fats	It is better to use mustard, til or sunflower oil for cooking. These contain unsaturated fat.
Spices and Condiments	No spices and condiments, etc. are Condiments allowed to the yogis as these have been found to be stimulating and to act as unwholesome irritants and are harmful. Similarly, highly seasoned stuffs, exciting and intoxicating drinks are prohibited.
Tea and Coffee	Tea and coffee are acidic. The practice of taking them immediately after major meals is bad. caffeine in coffee and tea is responsible for the stimulating effect. As far as possible, one should restrict it to only two cups a day.

The ideal food for man is the food which contributes to greater endurance, is revitalizing and health-promoting. It consists of grains, dairy products like milk, curd (yoghurt), buttermilk and cottage cheese, vegetables carrot and beetroot and lots of salad, fresh fruits, nuts, honey and nutritive roots.

11.4 QUANTITY OF FOOD

Moderation in diet (mitahara) is emphasised as the guideline- to eat no more or no less than what is absolutely necessary to satisfy one's appetite. Moreover, the yogis further believed in filling only half the stomach with food, a quarter with water and leaving the rest for fermentative gases or air.

11.5 WHEN TO EAT

Food should be taken only when hungry. A light breakfast and two principal meals (lunch and dinner) are considered sufficient for a person leading a sedentary life. Between the intervals of the principal meals, it is advisable not to eat anything. Each time there should be a four-hour gap between breakfast, lunch, evening tea and dinner. It is advisable that no water be taken with food, it checks digestion and such delays produce indigestion. The best thing is to take water half an hour before or after a meal.

11.6 HOW TO EAT

Masticate your food properly and learn to appreciate natural taste and flavour of fruits and vegetables. It will also lessen the chances of overeating.

Remember, according to Shri Yogendraji, "Impaired digestion results from taking into the body food wrongly selected in kind or in quantity, wrongly prepared or wrongly masticated."

Remember, always eat your liquids and drink your solids.

11.7 BALANCED DIET

A diet which provides all the necessary nutrients is called a Balanced diet. There are six basic elements of food which provide, what is called, a square meal. These meet an individual's needs in all known nutrients.

These in terms of natural foodstuffs are shown below as they should be included in your daily meals for good health and are grouped under 'A' and 'B' (Refer to chart).

A SQUARE MEAL

GROUP 'A' (Negative food) to supply warmth and energy to the body for growth and development.

Proteins	*Carbo-hydrates*	*Fats*
Cereals Milk & Milk products Legumes & pulses. Oilseeds & nuts. Soyabeans	Cereals Sugar Gur	Oil Butter Ghee Nuts

GROUP 'B' (Positive food) To give protection against disease and ill-health and to regulate body-functions

Vitamins	*Minerals*	*Water*
Citrus fruits, Green & yellow leafy vegetables. Salad greens	vegetables, Dry fruits	Safe, clean pure water

The foods that are healthful are distinguished as positive foods and come under Group B, and those that are negative come under Group A. 'Civilised' people eat more negative foods or foods in excess, neglecting the positive foods which are helpful in maintaining the normal working condition of the body. For a healthy person the formula of 2:1 (positive and negative) is recommended or 80 per cent and 20 per cent so that the glands and organs of the body function efficiently; helps in the peristaltic action of the intestines and eliminating waste matter; assist digestion and stimulate the nervous system.

Scientists are unanimous that over-nutrition through an excess of calories stored as fat can contribute materially to physical deterioration and quicken the ageing process. Consumption of more fats may cause obesity. And deposition of fat in the body under the skin and around organs like the heart is bad, with attendant risks of heart diseases and diabetes.

11.8 HOW TO GET THE BEST OUT OF FOOD

1. GREEN AND YELLOW VEGETABLES including carrot are mostly full of vitamin A. Spinach contains a lot of iron which we need for the haemoglobin in red blood corpuscles (RBCs). It can be better absorbed if it is taken together with vitamin C. For instance a dash of nimbu (lemon) on palak-ki-bhaji.

2. RAW VEGETABLES (Salads): Use raw vegetables made of chopped carrots, onions, raddish (moolee), cucumber, a little tomato and chutneys in which mint (pudina) is used.

3. VITAL GROUP OF 'B' VITAMINS: Hand-pounded rice, unpolished wheat, dals (pulses) and green leafy vegetables.

4. FERMENTATION: Fermentation is used everywhere in India in making curd, batter for dosa, idli etc. Fermentation multiplies the contents of vitamins several-fold, increases iron availability and greatly improves the digestibility of the starch and proteins in food.

5. VITAMIN 'C': Good and cheap sources of this vitamin are amla (Gooseberry), lemon juice and raw onion. The guava contains six times as much vitamin 'C' as six oranges, but one amla contains twice as much as guava. Remember vitamin 'C' is destroyed by cooking and exposure to sunlight.

   Sprouting or germination is a simple way o increasing the vitamin 'C' content and digestibility of many foodstuffs. Green gram - Phaseolus Radiatus (moong) germinated is very potent in vitamin 'C'.

   To sprout seeds at home, add water (one-half to an equal quantity) to the moong or Bengal gram and leave for 8 to 16 hours till fully absorbed. Tie the swollen grains in a muslin cloth, place on a plate and invert a wire bowl over it and allow to sprout for 12 to 24 hours.

6. PROTEIN: Soyabean flour contains 40 per cent protein; peas lentils and dried beans between 20 to 25 per cent. Use a little curd or buttermilk with each meal to boost the protein quantity.

7. VITAMIN 'D': It is found in cheese, curds and milk and all varieties of greens. There is plentiful sunshine all the year round. This vitamin is formed on the skin when exposed to sunlight, which is needed for strong bones and calm nerves. Strip and sunbathe your naked body for at least 15 minutes every morning or evening or wear white clothes, preferably khadi, when exposed to sunlight.

8. Replace tea or coffee with a decoction of tulsi leaves and ginger.

11.9 SOME IMPORTANT GUIDELINES

TAKE

- Low-salt diet or less of salt
- Low-fat dairy products and especially yoghurt and buttermilk.
- A generous helping of leafy and greens vegetables and fresh fruits everyday.
- Sprouted seeds should be included in the menu at least twice a week. These are rich in vitamins C,A,E,K and several of the B-Complex group.
- Take half a teaspoon of honey in your tea. It is rapidly and easily assimilated and is a heart and muscle stimulant.

AVOID

- Processed, refined sugar and synthetic foodstuffs.
- Eating snacks and other titbits constantly between meals.
- Fat, rich meat, pork, egg yolk, prawns and shellfish.
- White bread, strong tea, coffee, all types of condiments, tinned foods, biscuits and cakes, puddings, processed cheese, fried foods, soft drinks.
- Avoid the use of baking soda as it destroys vitamins.
- Drinking water while eating (or during meals).
- Deep-fried foods like pakoras, puris, samosa etc.
- Avoid aluminum utensils for cooking.

DO NOT

- Eat when you are not hungry.
- Eat when tired, angry or emotionally upset.
- Eat when you are having work immediately after meal.
- Eat foods containing colouring or flavouring agents.

DO

- Try to relax a little, after a day's hard work, before commencing your meal.
- Take plenty of time over your meal and masticate your food thoroughly.

REMEMBER

- Missing an evening meal once a week, will be beneficial.
- The risk factors in the development of coronary heart disease,

strokes, kidney disease and diabetes are:

1. overweight
2. high cholesterol levels
3. cigarette smoking
4. lack of exercise
5. hypertension

- Overeating and overweight go hand in hand, along with lack of exercise.
- One ounce of body fat equals about 219 calories. If you want to reduce, cut your calorie intake by 500 calories a day, you should lose about 1 pound a week or 4 pounds in a month. It is safe.
- Slimming foods can cause both physical and psychological damage.
- Vegetables should be baked, steamed or prepared in a pressure cooker. Food should not be overcooked.
- Food material should not be extremely hot, cold or excessively spiced.
- In any kind of abuse, be it in food, alcohol or tobacco, the body is the sufferer.

PART III

12

MIND: THE CAUSE OF BONDAGE AND RELEASE

12.1 PSYCHOSOMATIC PROBLEMS

Yoga shows the way out of the complexities and problems of life and holds the key to 'Better Living'. This has been amply proved by an intensive study of 116 cases in the management of psychiatric and psychosomatic disorders undertaken in 1971 by Yoga Institute, Santa Cruz, Bombay. The results were highly encouraging and an overall improvement of 77.58 per cent was recorded by the psychiatrist which, according to him, seemed to surpass the results of psychoanalytical therapy in various series.

There is a growing realization in the medical field that many of our diseases are psychosomatic, associated with mental and emotional disturbances. This realization dawned on the medical profession when it discovered a group of patients whose symptoms were quite definite, but in whom no organic cause of disease could be found. Fifty years ago, little was understood about this type of cases and patients were lumped together under the diagnosis of 'functional' or 'non-organic' disease - a vague classification. This did nothing to help the patient. After much research, the medical men found one factor common to nearly all these cases - a BACKGROUND OF ANXIETY and the vague term 'functional' was replaced by ANXIETY-state'. It is said that the present era is an age of Anxiety - the commonest form of psychoneurosis. But then it still remain a puzzle why so many different symptoms (resultant reactions) were produced by this anxiety state. There is a wide spectrum of anxiety of TENSION states including psychosomatic and organic illness with associated anxiety and physical tension.

A very simple form of ANXIETY REACTIONS displayed in normal

adaptation to environmental stress is one encountered by students before examinations or by one making a speech for the first time. Little more in intensity is the anxiety pertaining to worries about something specific like health, job, security, or sexual adequacy etc., i.e., reactions of a psychological nature. This could get aggravated further by unrecognized conflict and guilt - feeling of despair feeling of helplessness and hopelessness, utter confusion and unworthiness. All this may work up to a point where an impulsive individual thinks of suicide. Or, it may be a non-specific psychological type of anxiety - more constitutional, pertaining to an individual's personality.

It was also found that all functional cases in which patients were living under continual stimulus of fear or anxiety, give rise to certain common symptoms like palpitation of the heart, increased blood pressure, insomnia, tiredness, dysepsia etc. This persistent maladjustment often leads to aggravation of a physiological weakness which produces organic malfunctioning, or to a dysfunction in the autonomic nervous system which, in turn, constitutes a physical disease. What particular manner this psychological stress shows itself in somatic symptoms depends on which is the weakest organ in the system.

12.1.1 Emotional Stress can Cause Distressing Symptoms

But remember, there is an EMOTIONAL TONE of anxiety in all such cases giving rise to all kinds of abdominal distress. In fact, medical reports from the world over reveal that two-thirds of all patients seen by doctors, in both general and hospital practice, suffer from afflictions of which EMOTIONAL TENSION is the primary cause.

12.1.2 Emotionally-Induced Illness

EMOTIONS can upset glandular function and metabolic balance. Some of the other internal changes are in the rate of heart-beat, blood pressure, blood chemistry, rate of respiration, galvanic skin response and metabolic changes in brainwaves. All stomach distresses are emotional. In an angry man, the stomach soaks up blood like sponge, turns fiery red and splashes acid. In a man who is frightened, the stomach lies still and pale - blood vessels shrink and squeeze most of the blood out. During emotional stress - even the lining of the stomach wall, when observed through medical instruments, is seen to change its colour with different emotional stimuli. Some of the most commonly occurring symptoms due to emotional activity are: a constant feeling of tiredness, loss of appetite, insomnia, constipation, mood fluctuations with a feeling of uneasiness, palpitation, excessive sweating from palms and soles, and several gynaecological disorders in case of women. There is a growing awareness of the importance of emotional factors on both the activities and efficiency of the heart and circulatory system. It is all EMOTIONALLY-INDUCED ILLNESS as Doctor Johan A. Schindler, puts it. Under a hectic life of an industrialised society, a person under stress may characteristically become hypertense. A variety of stress-worry, lifelong conflicts over authority, repressed hostility, constant fatigue and so on - tighten artery walls or cause constriction of the blood vessels, and raise blood pressure. Stress and strain can contribute to rheumatic fever, to high blood pressure and eventually to heart attacks.

Another way of looking at this matter is that certain personality types are associated with such psychosomatic affection.

12.1.3 The Ulcer Personality

This is a psycho-physiologic gastro-intestinal reaction. It is said that a feeling of strong resentment, sustained hostility and anxiety (by parasympathetic overcompensation) results in a perceptible increase of acid production (HCL) which eats away away the stomach lining or the lining of the duodenum, leaving a kind of wound. And this anxiety is often intensified by a sense of responsibility associated with being in authority as in case of ambitious driving individuals - like business executives or successful tycoons.

12.1.4. The Asthma Personality

This is a psycho-physiological respiratory reaction to certain oppressing life situations (innervation to the lungs through the parasympathetic nervous system). The mucous cells are induced to secrete and there is marked vasodilation of the blood vessels with swelling of tissues. In short, the air-ways become congested and breathing becomes difficult. Hypersensitive, insecure individuals, afraid of losing love and protection or having difficulties in obtaining the needed love and support, are generally victims of this anxiety-borne disease.

Dr. Meyer Friedman, cardiovascular research director at Mount Zion Hospital, San Francisco, contends that men with certain personality traits such as individuals who have 'free floating hostility', insecurity, tendency of looking at everything as a challenge and who are addicted to habit formulations, are more prone to heart attacks (coronary disease).

12.2 STRESS DISEASES EXPRESSED IN PSYCHO-PHYSIOLOGICAL REACTION

The psychosomatic diseases are now called by the name of STRESS DISEASES expressed by psycho-physiological reactions and these problems are very much linked up with personality patterns. The example we had given was the ulcer personality where the person has psycho-physiologic gastro-intestinal reaction to life situation or with the Asthmatic personality, it is the psycho-physiologic respiratory reaction to life situation. To understand the problem more clearly we can say there is the interplay of three factors, as shown in the following diagram:

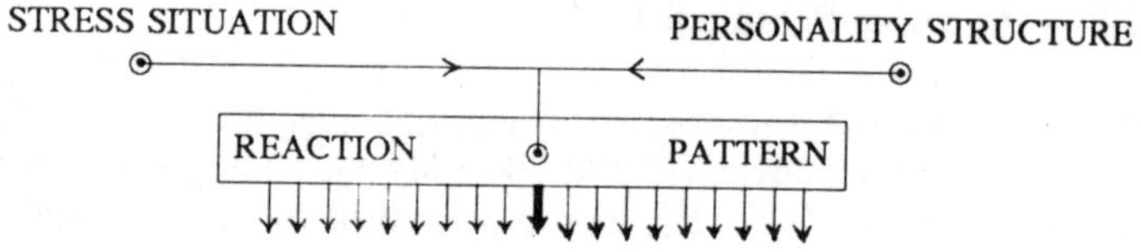

Stress condition of 'X' intensity
Expressed in terms of worry anxieity depression, fear etc.

Your individual personality complex, in meeting any oppressing stress situation, creates within you a reaction pattern in terms of worry, anxiety, fear, depression etc., resulting in STRESS CONDITION of 'X' intensity. Why 'X' intensity? Because it is going to differ from person to person. Even situations which cause tension to one individual may not cause any tension in another person. Stress produces its effect upon the body through the pituitary and the adrenal glands as they equip the body to the tremendous task of flight or fight. Over-stimulation of the endocrine glands and the nervous system results in impairment of physiological functioning expressed in terms of malfunctioning of some part or organ - whichever is the weakest in the individual organism. It is the weaker link which always gives way. Aided by new biochemical techniques and a vastly-expanded understanding of immunology and neurochemistry, the fast growing field of research and studies, shows that emotions acting through the brain, can affect:

(i) The nervous system
(ii) The hormone levels
(iii) The immunological responses

This changes the individual's susceptibility to a host of organic illnesses. A strong mind-body linkage is now proved once and for all and that has put to rest the Cartesian dichotomy that has separated body and mind since the 17th century. Dr. George F. Solomon, University of California psychiatrist said: "Mind and body are inseparable. The brain influences all sorts of physiological processes that were once thought not being centrally regulated." With the increasing concern over the "STRESS EPIDEMIC" in the U.S.A., numerous new fields have sprung up: behavioural medicine to battle stress-related illness, psychoneuroimmunology - to explore the way EMOTIONAL STATES affect the body's defences, etc. Furthermore, a person under stress takes a longer time to heal from a given disease than does a person not so situated. The process of ageing is also accelerated under conditions of stress.

In any case, prolonged stress (Mental and Emotional) in any form plays an important part in the development and final outcome of almost any disease of the body, be it common cold or cancer. If we examine, stress is generally involved in loss or threat to individual status, goals, health, job, security etc. There are different forms of stresses in day-to-day life. Some of the STRESS-PRODUCING EVENTS are:

(a) **Death**: Death of spouse or of a close relative,marital separation, divorce, marriage etc.

(b) **Home**: Trouble with in-laws, family conflict and tension, illness, sickness etc. in family, even change in living condition etc.

(c) **Office**: Trouble with boss, inability to handle subordinates, losing job, business readjustment, change in financial status etc.

So there are different forms of stresses in day-to-day life. Under the conditions of worry and anxiety, overwork, fatigue and chronic infections, some people, even if they pull on for sometime, break down with different diseases, either singly or in combination. Some get high blood pressure, others hardening of the blood vessels and coronary heart disease, and yet others rheumatoid arthritis etc.

12.2.1 Internally Generated Pressure

Yoga was the first system in the world to recognize the connection and the interaction between the body and the mind. It tells you that mind influences the body much more than the body influences the mind, a fact which is clearly witnessed in psychosomatic and psychiatric disorders. An important thing to remember is that stress is measured and evaluated in terms of how it is experienced by the person himself or, in other words, what the event means to that person. It is when a person fails to adjust to his emotional or psychological conflicts, and the STRESS is prolonged and far exceeds the level of TOLERANCE, that a person develops what can be called as CRITICAL STRESS, and if he CANNOT COPE with it, then either the mind or the body has to break down and that is when–

STRESS ⟶ leads to ⟶ DISTRESS

An interesting feature of the medical study report, 1971, of the research unit of The Yoga Institute, Santa Cruz Bombay, referred to earlier in this chapter, was that most of the patients had not had much of external STRESS. The problems mainly had arisen from internal stresses caused by conflicts and complexes in relation to the self. It is all INTERNALLY GENERATED PRESSURE. One has to understand the sources of STRESS and TENSION within an individual. These causes of restlessness and tension are often deeply embedded in our life-style and our PERSONALITY COMPLEX - our thinking, feeling, temperament, disposition, basic values and attitudes. Most of the 'pressure' comes from within ourselves. Situations which cause tension to one individual may not cause the same tension in others. It seems it is not the situation but ourselves who have to take the blame. We seem to be aware of tension only at the level of its symptoms rather than its causes. The symptoms appear at the site of the organ but the cause generally lies elsewhere in the subtle body and in the YOGA SENSE, this cause lies in the CHITTA - the PERSONALITY-COMPLEX. What is significant in a stress condition is that "the degree of mental and emotional stress produced in an individual going through a STRESS-producing situation depends to a large extent on how he or she is habituated to REACT TO IT." "This is important irrespective of the situation and the profession." Yoga tries to re-educate the patient to alter his habitual reaction pattern, develop a coping mechanism and thus holds the key to better living. Yoga has laid down psycho-somatic means through various psycho-physiological processes for dealing with the body-mind complex. It tries to harmonise and integrate the human personality at all levels and stages of life.

Shri Yogendraji says: "Yoga suggests an integrated approach to man with the personality-complex (Chitta) as the basic factor and treats man as a body-mind complex."

The future physician has to be such who will not only treat the disease at the symptomatic level but also handle the personality-complex in its psychic factor, restoring harmony to the whole personality of the patient.

2.3 THE PERSONALITY COMPLEX (CHITTA)

Man is what his mind is.' - Shri Yogendraji

In defining mind, yoga has adopted a broad concept. It defines it beautifully by the monosyllabic word "Chitta" - a compound of many things. That truly represents the total psychological make-up of an individual. It consists of our ego, intellect (buddhi), mind (manas), senses and the root or source potentials of samskarvasana from the soul's past experience i.e., impressions and tendencies lying dormant either racial, hereditary, autogenic or otherwise. What emerges as the sum total of all these is the PERSONALITY COMPLEX which is the true meaning of CHITTA. For the modern psychologists, the concept of personality is of rather recent origin. In trying to find the mind as an entity, the Applied psychologists lost it in the way and have now replaced it with the new word - Concept of behaviour.

The point to remember is that each self (purusha) is associated with or possessed of a special "chitta" and, therefore, there are infinite "chittas" with infinite beings suffering from pain (dukha) which are symptoms of anarchy, imperfection and disquietude due to *emotional conflicts* and *tension,* inhibiting an individual from any real progress toward self-evolution. Reactions vary under different circumstances or at different times, with different people. Why are there different reactions? The reason is that since each individual has a different "chitta" of his/her own so different resultant reactions are produced by even the same kind of anxiety-state. Yoga ideology and technology, through its various psycho-physiological processes, deal with the body-mind complex and tries to harmonise and integrate the human personality. Disciplining of human personality complex (Chitta) and its integration is the first essential to live fully and achieve the best.

12.3.1 Personality Complex and its Components

EGO	Ahamkara - the sense of 'I' - ness
INTELLECT	Buddhi
MIND	Manas: Analytical mechanism or coordinating organ which janalyses and synthesises somewhat like a computer.
SENSES	Faculties of receiving sensation, general or particular, through various senses etc.
ROOT POTENTIALS	Root potentials, tendencies lying dormant deep into the recesses of the subconscious - the unknown part of man.

12.4 FUNDAMENTAL CAUSE OF HUMAN MISERY AND SUFFERING

The fundamental cause of all human misery and suffering lies in the philosophy of *Kleshas* (affliction) propounded by Patanjali. The *kleshas* function through the personality-complex, constituting the psychomental stream of our daily life.

There are five *kleshas*, namely: (i) ignorance, (ii) egoism, (iii) attachment, (iv) aversion and (v) clinging to life. These are the underlying causes of the *karmas* we generate by our thoughts, desires and actions, binding ourselves in the karma cycle of birth, life, suffering, death and rebirth.

Ignorance (avidya) of one's real self, is the main cause - the breeding ground - and the other four *kleshas* follow in a chain. It is the false knowledge, mistaking the non-eternal for the eternal, the unpleasant for the pleasant and the non-self for the self.

The next element which further compounds this ignorance is the ego - complications begin since it is this very element that gives rise to the factor of personality - the sense of supreme importance of 'I'. It is a real anti-spiritual aspect in man.

According to Ramana Maharshi, the chief obstacle to the realization of the self is this 'I', which creates the illusion of a separate individuality. His method was of self-inquiry (Atma-vichara), and 'Who am I'? He says "Ultimately, *sadhana* is simply an attack on the ego and no amount of ecstasy or meditation can carry it to success so long as the ego remains entrenched in hope and fear, ambition and resentment, in any sort of passion or desire."

Once individuality gets established, resulting in wrong identification of the ego, the man gets caught in the ever-expanding desire-complex to gain name, fame and power. The personality is the person 'I'-ego (ahamkara). Ego, the very cause of all evil, is now getting recognised through yoga by advanced Western thinkers also. Man starts working on the ego defence mechanism, whenever there is a threat to the integrity or worth of this 'I', which, according to James C. Coleman, is a high degree of self-deception and reality-distortion and comes very much in the way of adjustment problems. He says, "The integrating core of the personality is built up on ego involvement, and any threat to the self shall arouse anxiety; consequently, the psychiatric patient would try to build up various defence mechanisms around the self which is called into play in any stress situation resulting in reaction formation."

From egoism springs desire or attachment which has two main expressions: Attraction (raga) and Repulsion (dvesa). Attraction is for pleasurable experiences resulting in attachment to them. Repulsion is to avoid contact with any object which has previously inflicted pain. These two cover the entire range of sensation and emotional experience and we are caught up in the play of the opposites which creates likes and dislikes. We collect and build up a paraphernalia of objects for enjoyment and undergo a fear-complex for their loss.

The final result of all feelings and emotion is love for life (abhinivesa) or clinging to life and fear of death, knowing fully well that we have to make the final exit whether we are kings or commoners. While commenting on this, Vyasa argues that the presence of this *klesha* implies the existence of a previous life. Since the desire to perpetuate life and a fear of impending death is seen present in all, it is concluded that the experience of death in a previous existence is the root of the fear of death in this life as well. These five *kleshas* collectively form the nature and content of experiences of an infinite variety and leave a trace of potency (samskar) in the *chitta* which serves as a great storehouse of all past experiences. These in turn ripen and produce one life after another in a never-ending cycle according to the law of cause and effect which pervades the universe. The individual is merely born with a body, a mind, a character and social surroundings which express, as it were, the sum-total of his *karmic* balance at that particular moment of time.

12.4.1 Summary

To summraise, the *chitta* wanders through the senses and is affected and ruffled by desires, hatred, egoistic attachment and passion which shatter one's peace and happiness. The result is that most of the time one is captivated or overcome by stimuli and lets oneself be helplessly swept away in a mere reaction to them. The pleasant captivates one's mind and one reacts with liking it and runs after further pleasant experiences and ultimately one is caught in the craze for sensual pleasures. To the unpleasant, one reacts by disliking it and wants to get away from it or be rid of it. That means one reacts not to the situation as such but to the situation as one evaluates it especially in relation to one's feelings. Besides, there may be conflict between what is and what should be, or confusion of values and one is not able to resolve this. If one has developed a little deeper understanding, one will know that one's mind is engaged most of the time in egocentric activities, a false sense of identification, which brings in the sense of possession and there seems to be no end to one's ambitions and material aspirations. In short, in this complex web, one lives a life of perpetual conflict, tension and anxiety. The *kleshas* can be got rid off by the practice of yoga, they need not deter anyone from taking to the study and practice of yoga. What is more significant to an aspirant of yoga are the obstacles - physical and mental - that he faces in his life itself. They are enumerated by Patanjali as sickness, idleness, doubt, carelessness, sloth, lack of detachment, misapprehension, non-achievement of a stage of concentration, and inability to stay in that stage of concentration.

Now this *chitta* (personality-complex) has received utmost attention in yoga technology (sadhana patha) since it is believed that if the individual can discipline, control the *chitta*, the whole problem will get automatically solved.

According to Patanjali, there are five states of the *chitta.*

12.4.2 Five States of Chitta

Ksipta	: Distracted or disintegrated, extreme restless state when the mind has many emotional conflicts and longings.
Mudha	: Diffused, infatuated and forgetful, this state tends towards ignorance, sleep and lethargy.
Viksipta	: Occasionally steady.
Ekagra	: Concentrated, devoted to a single object.
Niruddha	: A restrained or controlled mind. The yogi belongs to this category.

This clearly shows that steadiness of *chitta* has to be achieved - that undisturbed calmness of the flow of mind which, truly speaking, is the central feature of all yoga practices. Now how can one reach this state? By the destruction of the impurities that exist in the *chitta* and by sustaining an attitude of detachment (vairagya). Patanjali defines yoga as the control of the thought-waves of the *chitta.*

'Yoga chitta vritti nirodhah.'

Each individual is a bundle of sensations, thoughts and ideas which are always in a state of flux. *Chitta,* which is a subtle substance of matter, always exists in the form of its states which are called *vrittis*. It undergoes modifications and this has to be stopped and controlled and then alone will the *chitta* be able to come in contact with the pure consciousness. Abiding in this state will give you lasting peace and supreme happiness by destroying all *kleshas*. It can further lead you on to perfection and the highest discriminative knowledge (prajna) which will dispel all ignorance.

"It is the purpose of Yoga to free the personality complex from the bondage of thoughts, feelings and reflexes which have accumulated in the subconscious. The balanced mind or intellect is possible only then," says Shri Yogendraji.

Remember: Yoga is basically a way of life which has been evolved as a system to go beyond the personality-complex and achieve liberation (kaivalya) - absolute freedom - liberation of soul from the matter.

PART IV

13

GUIDELINES FOR SELF-UNDERSTANDING

13.1 INTRODUCTION

The average man takes to the study and practice of yoga for the basic requirement of physical and psychomental fitness to get a feeling of total well-being. Some practise yoga with the expectation to improve various mental faculties like thinking, memory, judgement and concentration for a sharp and alert mind, some to enjoy the benefits of deep relaxation and meditation. A very small percentage vaguely wants an experience of a spiritual type. Therefore, there are grades of people and grades of achievements. But the basic foundation of success in yoga rests on two primary factors.

1. *Abhyasa* : habituation to practice with perseverance and patience.
2. *Vairagya*: Dispassion or mental quality of detachment from external influences and from all types of distractions.

13.1.1 How Yoga Operates

According to Shri Yogendraji — yoga accessories (8-fold path) operate in two directions, viz., (i) in dissociating the impurities (viyogakarana) and (ii) in removing the obstacles which obstruct the course of mind for attaining the desired perfection (Aptikarana). Keeping in mind the higher objectives in yoga some important guidelines on living have been laid down which will help you to solve your psychosomatic problems or will guard you against such diseases, which are on the increase in big cities. It will grant you sedate and positive health, happiness and peace of mind. When pursued with due intensity and singleness of purpose, it can bring about a qualitative change in the personality-complex and can make way for psychic unfoldment.

13.2 THE PSYCHOMENTAL STREAM OF LIFE

According to our central doctrine and belief, the law of *karma* is operative in physical world applicable to one and all which is the natural sequence of cause and effect closely linked up with the cycle of birth, death and rebirth. Evolution, therefore, is a cyclic process. In this journey towards evolution each individual soul (Purusha), under the bondage of this law of *karma* is simply reborn in an environment and surrounding which is best suited for it, carrying with it a sort of *prakritic* reservoir (accumulated *karmasaya* of endless lives) in seed form deep down in our *chitta*, in the subconscious part of our personality-complex. It is this *karmasaya* as the limiting factor which ripens into life state, (Janam and Jati), span of life (ayush) and life-experience (Bhoga), pleasurable or painful (the karmic suffering). In other words, this karmic suffering and the fruits of karma are properly distributed for each one of us and it is there to serve the inherent purpose of liberation, whether we are conscious of it or not.

13.2.1 Yoga Psychology

Each individual, endowed with a special *chitta* by a particular combination of the *gunas* (sattva, rajas and tamas), is merely born with a body, a mind, a character and social surroundings which express, as it were, the sum total of his *karmic* balance at that particular moment of time. This chitta has a structural defect of afflictions (*kleshas*), namely, ignorance, egosim, attraction and repulsion and clinging to life. The functioning of these kleshas through the personality-complex results in infinite waves of mental activity (*chitta-vriti*), the variable and ever-changing world of desires, perception, thoughts, feelings constituting the psychomental stream of our daily life.

It is important to note that whichever way the chitta functions it creates trouble unless and until the *kleshas* or afflictions and the resulting karmas and the age-old *vasana* (residual desire potencies) are all burnt up by the *viveka* (fire of discrimination). So when the entire thinking process of chitta starts from the *Prajna* (wisdom side) and not the *klesha* side, then alone the human being is free from pain and suffering. The *kleshas* are at the back of what are called *karmasaya* (vehicle of actions) — a sort of spring board. The philosophy of kleshas forms the foundation of the yogic philosophy — it is thus an analysis of the underlying and fundamental cause of human misery and suffering. These *kleshas* form a connected series of causes and effects and involve us in a never-ending cycle of births and deaths and miseries of life and the entire process of *karma* cycle. Patanjali is more concerned about the powerful desire complex and the ego around which the psychomental stream of life revolves. The *chitta* becomes an arena of all our conflicts, urges, fears, impulses, tendencies and dispositions and works compulsively upon us from within. This creates great hindrances in our real progress towards a peaceful and harmonious living. Our chitta which truly represents the psychological inner make-up of our personality with the ego and the desire complex complicates the matter so that everything in our life and world, we measure from the ego point of view. Ego-Apamkara is the real anti-spiritual aspect in Man — the egocentric individual desires that events should follow his plan and that he knows better not only of events but of the individuals. He, therefore, expects the world to move around his own ideas. "If I cannot exist, there is no room for you with me." In actual fact, the world moves not according to individual idea but according to certain laws that prevail. Ego does not know or recognize it, and as a result it suffers tremendous pain. From egoism springs the desire of attachment which has two main expressions — Attraction and Repulsion.

(i) Desire to attract, in order to possess or again to come into contact with any object which has previously afforded pleasure.
(ii) Desire to repel, in order to drive far away or to avoid contact with any object which has previously inflicted pain.

This attachment and aversion covers the entire range of sensational and emotional experience — the two together forming a pair of opposite reaction patterns:

ATTRACTION — a driving towards
REPULSION — a driving away

and these are the two great motor energies in life into which all desires are ultimately resolvable.

The self comes under the bondage of desire — of attraction and repulsion, and is attracted hither and thither, repelledfrom this or that, hurried about among pleasures of pains and pains of pleasure-giving objects, as a helmless ship — undirected, vague and groping. The more one steps into these *kleshas*, the greater the disturbance of the chitta, resulting in greater mistakes in judgement. This state also leads to what is called *PRAJNA-APRADHA*. The final result of feelings and emotion is love of life — *Abhinivesa* — the strong desire for life which dominates even the learned or the wise persons. The reaction pattern is not objective or discriminative — it is confused by feelings. This false identification is not considered superficially by Patanjali but rather he goes into great detail in the depth study of personality-complex. The whole yoga technology is very much laid down to discipline and to mould the chitta or personality-complex to meet highest emotional or intellectual pattern and finally to transcend personality-complex to gain kavalya or real freedom.

13.3 GREATEST THREAT TO PEACE AND HAPPINESS OF HUMANITY

Modernism, with its emphasis on materialism and sensuous culture, has brought in a lot of artificiality where the stress is on quantity rather than on quality. Worldly values dominate the creature man, reacting to stimuli, struggling for self-preservation, self-aggrandizement and self-gratification; permissive hedonistic society has brought human values to mere sensory, material things —which has inspired anti-social and destructive forms of behaviour and relationships. Moreover, there are forces of propaganda and brainwashing right from the manufacturers to politicians. In youth, there is clear evidence of unrest and frustration, all the world over, arising from a materialistic outlook on life and freedom from moral restraint, leading to a crisis of character at all levels. With the idea that repression or suppression is bad, freedom is given, drugs are taken excessively which later on become an addiction and an obsession. Religion is at a discount and the current educational system does not seem to have any ennobling effect whatsoever. All this constitutes the greatest threat to the life, peace and happiness of humanity.

The modern man, therefore, does need to be re-educated, as it were, to enable him to find the basis of a healthy, creative and satisfying life. His various inner faculties and resources have to be mobilized to serve his best interests by elevating his consciousness and by giving him lasting success and true happiness with a faith in a supersensible reality.

Yoga education as a way of life can transform the individual, social and national character and the outlook of youth and help to bring into being a better society for tomorrow. It integrates human personality for a fuller and richer life that alone can aim at the highest and achieve the best.

13.3.1 Discipline or Corruption

Man is said to be the supreme product, the crowning achievement of Nature. Of course, the laws of gravitation and biological selection are common to both man and animal. But what distinguishes man from an animal is that he has a superior intelligence to discriminate and a free will to act. He can defy and even break the set pattern of behaviour and can check the wayward impulse of desire, impose discipline and control himself.

Man, therefore, stands in between the two alternatives: Discipline and Corruption, and he has to choose but one. It is said, "No man can serve two masters; either he can serve God or the Devil."

Corruption is corroding the soul and killing your conscience. Repetitive acts of such nature make you thick-skinned and you lose completely your awareness of the subconscious mind which keeps on sending reminder after reminder till you become dead to all such inner signals. Nature then takes its own course of teaching and you have to pay the price in the end. All this may be a very gradual frustrating experience unless you become wiser after each such lapse on your part and change your sense of values, thinking, attitude, habit structure and way of life.

13.3.2 Yamaniyama — The First Two Steps

According to yoga man is in a process of evolution, he has still certain urges, animal nature, instincts, basic, emotions tinted by the impurities of his personality complex. In the ultimate analysis, the ancient yogis came to the conclusion that the mind has got to be disciplined, controlled and made steady. For this, a certain attitude of mind is to be developed, some acclimatization to moral living was absolutely necessary for a healthy and balanced life. The first two steps of Yamaniyama in yoga are a disciplinary process relating to the integral conditioning of the body-mind complex which determines the personal attitude and behaviour, first towards oneself and then towards the society, In our character, the subjective value of action is stressed since "EVERY ACTION IS AN OUTER EXPRES-

SION OF THE INNER MAN." There lies the possibility of his overcoming the animality in him, becoming human and growing into Divinity —rising from his ignoble traits to noble.

According to Shri Yogendraji, "The impure, diffused, distracted and disintegrated mind is a great personal impediment standing in the way of individual and social well-being." Sadhana-applied yoga has founded the technology to purify and integrate the personality complex at all levels of life.

13.3.3 Five Yamas: Conditioned Yoga Behaviour

Yamas condition man's behaviour, both personal and social. Let us consider these five yamas. The gate to yoga is through self-restraint. Keeping the mind most of the time in an unmodified condition — *vritti-Nirodha* is the keynote —restraining the mental modification and making the mind steady is the Central feature of all yoga practices.

AHIMSA (Non-violence): Don't injure or hurt others. Ahimsa, like the footprint of an elephant which is so big that it envelops the footprints of all the other animals, is the greatest of all five yamas. It is regarded as mother of all virtues and on an analysis one finds, in a way, it envelops all the remaining yamas. Yoga does not believe in surface treatment. It catches us at the level of impulse and tells us that it is not only the physical action that matters but we should not even think of abusing or harming the other person. Thoughts and feelings also subtly affect others, the important thing here is intention — the state of mind. Are we violent? Are we angry? In our interaction with family members, relatives and friends, we must observe our hatred, our habits, our reactions. Our son or daughter has disobeyed and we feel we are getting angry for his or her good only but what actually happens is that we simply feel insulted, our ego is hurt because they have disobeyed. We have to analyse, go deep into our reaction and find out. Our anger, jealousy and greed will gradually get rooted out if we practice non-violence as we have to be kind and harmless in our thoughts, words and our deeds. In other words, *Ahimsa* demands a spirit of friendliness towards all creatures, a positive unselfish love for all. Mahatma Gandhi recognised non-violence as a basic virtue and applied it to the welfare of the humanity.

SATYA (Truth): Do not speak untruth. Untruth also means injury to others as it interferes with the legitimate rights of others. What we find is that often we lie to cheat — often inadvertently and sometimes consciously. Dishonesty is an affirmation of ego. The modern man is too selfish, he wants to succeed in the world and so he would not mind harming others by telling lies as long as it serves his purpose. In our everyday life and in our inter personal relationship at home, in office, in business, we see dishonesty and falsehood. This becomes a source of degradation of our own personality. In fact, speaking truth should be normal in human relationship, for without that we shall never succeed in our friendship and gaining social confidence. Telling lies is a breach of trust linked up with an element of cowardice. If we have spoken one lie, to hide it we have to speak ten lies, bringing unnecessary complications in life. We distort things or we convey or report or interpret events incorrectly. Truth becomes a casualty, facts are distorted or mixed up with one's own colouration of mind or if one is careless the real fact is not conveyed. It gives rise to a sense of guilt in our sub-conscious mind leading to stress conditions. The only exception is that truth which causes hurt or injury to another's feelings or which can cause harm to anyone is to be avoided, e.g., if one points out a wrong direction to a robber running after a person carrying money. In such situations one has to be discreet; means and ends have to be considered.

ASTEYA (non-stealing) and *APARIGRAH* (Non-covetousness): Do not take things which are not yours and desist from such acts as stealing. Stealing somebody's privilege or credit and any idea of misappropriation even in thoughts constitute a breach of Asteya. One can take only what legitimately belongs to him. Even taking more than what we need and then wasting it, is a form of stealing from the rest of mankind. Asteya and Aparigrah together constitute a social remedy for human greed and selfishness.

BRAHMACHARYA (Non-indulgence in sex): It is wrongly implied that disciplinary yoga is against marriage. The restraint in yoga in fact is not against marriage as such but against the misuse of sex whether in or out of marriage. Indisciplined sex has a corrosive effect on man in all aspects of life. Sex has created wars in the world and has ruined families. Sublimation of the bodily energy gives power, vigour, and resists fatigue and disease. Being unchaste is to be violent.

The question here is not so much about the value of discipline. These *yamas* are necessary in the interest of the individual and the society as all the vices arising out of lack of their observance end in violence. One may find that some yamas are easier and others are hard to follow. But at least make a beginning with any of these, whichever one considers easier, and observe it in all sincerity.

Remember restraint is the gateway to yoga. According to yoga, these five *yamas* guard us against the pitfalls to be avoided, and it is at every stage of impulse (pratyaya), when the individual is about to think, feel, speak or act that yoga takes charge and asks you to restrain against thinking, speaking or acting in a manner as would create complications.

13.3.4 Five Niyamas: Attitude Sublimated to Yoga Norms

SAUCA (Absolute purity): It covers not only cleanliness of the body and of the internal organs in the physical sense, but much more. It includes mental cleanliness and purity. A yogi lives in the world, mixes with the people and yet he is unaffected. The classic example given in this context is of the lotus leaf which remains dry though it is constantly in water.

SANTOSHA (Contentment): Since a yogi desires to hurt none, with no desire to speak untruth, no desire for lust and greed, he is perfectly satisfied and feels contented. If man is satisfied it means he has no desire or conversely if a man has no desire, he is satisfied.

TAPA (Fortitude): It points out more to a mental quality where a man remains undisturbed by opposide conditions — joy and sorrow, pleasure and pain, love and hatred etc. For the common man, avoiding indulgence and observing sense-control, proper food, yogic physical exercises for the body care and its improvement, acquiring calmness of mind and sublimation of emotions, constitute tapa and develop his will-power.

SVADHYAYA (Self-Study): It includes a disciplined study of self, nature and also scriptures and religious literature. Constant self-inquiry, introspection and awareness of painful and non-painful (Klishta or Aklishta) tendencies is very desirable for the student in order to evaluate his progress towards the Divine path. It also includes learning the laws of nature and a study of religious scriptures which gives him an insight into higher life. Practice of Japa of a Mantra, repetition of the sacred syllable 'AUM' is a part of Svadhyaya for divine communion.

ISHVARAPRANIDHANA (Resignation to the Will of the Absolute): It implies devotion or surrender to God and resignation to His Will. Submitting ourselves to the will of God is the only alternative left when tragedies or calamities engulf us. At that time, no argument and reasoning are to be resorted to, for this acts as a great psychological safety-valve which is bequeathed to the humanity in the face of sad situations.

Tapa, Svadhyaya and Ishvarpranidhana correspond to the triple nature of a human being related to his will, intellect and emotions respectively. It is regarded as Kriya yoga and is greatly recommended for the yoga aspirant.

Remember *Niyamas* deal with Attitude training, which is extremely vital for inner self-development.

13.4 LEARN TO UNDERSTAND YOURSELF

Objective: To know your Habitual Reaction Pattern

In the study of self-improvement, the first step is the awareness or becoming conscious of our body, working of the mind and all that is happening to us within and without. This habit of inner awareness has to start from the simple, gross level of the body, for example, when we are asked to sit in a meditative posture with our back straight and its broader application in day-to-day life is that we become conscious of our posture while sitting on a chair, standing or walking. How important is this for those having a faulty posture? It is by this habit of awareness that we will be able to read the body signals correctly and locate various factors that affect us in health and sickness. For minor ailments, we become our own doctor. A good way to develop awareness at the mental level is by getting into the habit of watching our reaction pattern to things, objects, persons, situations and events.

Life is made up of many things—joys and sorrows, moments of success and achievements, failures and disappointments, hopes, doubts and fear and moments of inspiration or depression and despair. Some people receive more than their share of troubles, trials, and tribulations, and life to them is a harsh competition, a cruel mockery, a world of pessimism.

If we observe carefully we find that, a great deal of our daily life is made up of small pinpricks, annoyances and perplexities. Many a time, we are carried away by emotions — the feeling part of our personality. Often we realise after we have spoken something or committed certain actions that we should not have said or behaved in such a manner. Common day-to-day occurrences in our family life would reveal how we get terribly upset, angry and lose our temper so easily. The servant perhaps has broken a piece of saucer of a newly-bought crockery set and the housewife flares up. She really gets angry. She could express her feelings in a quiet but firm tone, telling him to be extra careful in future. But to get really angry is to create an earthquake within which produces injurious chemical reactions in our system. Not able to locate an important paper or may be the car key at the right moment, missing a bus or train when there is urgency, unnecessary delay in waiting in the queue, less or more salt in the food during meals, heated arguments with our friend or business partner, between husband and wife are common examples of how we lose our patience or become impulsive. All these mental states and emotions not only create a disturbance in our mind but also affect our body, expressed as physiological tension and reactions as mentioned earlier. Often, we may experience a mental disturbance without knowing what its cause might be — maybe it is due to unconscious conflict or certain complexes pertaining to our individual personality. We have to recognise these problems and identify the factors which cause the tension by continual watch and self-analysis. Then alone, gradually we shall be able to find out how our mind works and what really is disturbing us. Our traits, our disposition, temperament, our attitude — all these factors contribute to it. The objective behind this is to change our habitual reaction pattern and by cultivating this habit of CONSTANT INTERNAL SELF-AWARENESS, we acquire a better understanding and a better control over our personality.

13.5 BHAVANA (Reflection)

Daily practice of *Bhavana* (Reflections)—Duration 10 minutes

The best way to do this practice is at night before you go to bed. Sit in Sukhasana or Vajrasana and recollect the happenings of the day or the previous day right from the time when you got up, through the morning, afternoon, evening and till bedtime. Try not to miss any detail. While you recall the event, consider the thoughts and feelings that went with the event. Make a special note of your actions and reactions to objects, persons and situations. Try to remember any desire not satisfied, any unpleasant situation or thing that spontaneously created a feeling of depression (if you are weak) or revolt (if you are strong). Note your emotional reactions and things that disturbed your mind, what things you left half done, promises you could not keep. In this practice of Bhavana — the journey to self-awareness — you have simply to sit back and let your mind watch your actions and reactions — you do not have to be critical about your shortcomings and weaknesses. In course of time, it will help integrate an objective attitude in life. At least you will be able to pass over the trivial annoyances of life. It will help you to change your habitual reaction pattern by watching constantly your thoughts, actions and behaviour.

13.6 PURUSHARTH (Motivation)

Objective: To understand your motives that move you

Yoga begins with the education of man through the process of awareness of his real motivations in life. This integrated training in the scientific yoga education in 'Better Living', is capable of providing us an ideal harmonious growth whch can surely strengthen and integrate our personality. Obviously, the first thing is to know ourselves as we are. "Know thyself" is still the key to wisdom as it was in the days of Socrates. Look to yourself and think about yourself. But we find the modern educated man with his very busy schedule in his life of hurry and worry, has minimal time to think about himself. He treats his body as he pleases and very often transgresses the rules of personal hygiene. There is misuse and abuse of his various senses. He is caught up in the play of the opposites and is not able to discriminate between essentials and non-essentials, good and really profitable. His value judgement seems to be poor. The ultimate result is that he finds himself a victim of endless mental conflicts, with his perception distorted and his judgement warped. Like a rudderless ship, he is carried away and drifts in the current of life by every gush of temptation, worry, frustation and disillusionment.

But supposing we are really dissatisfied and find life unsatisfactory at various levels and are willing to improve upon and do something about it. The first step is that we have got to think. First I am, then I think, I feel, I perceive, and then I act. Man is said to be the supreme product, the crowning achievement of nature. Of course, the laws of gravitation and biological selection are common to both man and animal. But what distinguishes man from an animal is his superior intelligence to discriminate and his free will to act. He can defy and even break the set pattern of behaviour (SR-bond) and check the wayward impulse of desire — impose discipline on and control himself. Human mind can think in many dimensions and is not carried away by instinct alone. He is a thinking-feeling personality. In fact, man is superior to his personality-complex which he can mould or discipline to meet his highest emotional or intellectual pattern.

So, we see that man develops purposely, distinctly and tries to establish his aims and objectives. Activity is the very essence of life. We call this PURUSHARTHA, translated as MOTIVATION, which means human effort. But motivations are of various types. A child going to the playground or a man going to the hospital to see his sick friend or a man going to post-office provide examples of immediate motivations. There are innumerable variables of these different types of motivations presenting a complex picture. But there are motivations which are deep and which guide our life. Our ancient seers and yogis have reduced these into four broad categories which give a basic picture about the total motivations, to bring about clarity in our thinking pertaining to our activity. Your each action is motivated by and can be reduced to these four factors DHARMA, ARTHA, KAMA and MOKSHA. These four major motivations have been given greater interpretation, in the modern terms of psychology, by the founder of the Yoga Institute — Shri Yogendraji. Though the meanings of these terms appear to be a little different in their synthesis, these arehaving the same import as their original meaning. We must remember that all real yoga is applied yoga and it must be translated in terms of living — in terms of ACTIONS. We are analysing actions and the attempt is to understand the real motivation behind each act of ours.

1. *DHARMA*: Literally it means 'what holds together.' This is generally translated as religion or in Buddhism it is called the Truth. Here Dharma means NATURAL RESPONSIBILITIES or/and DUTIES. Duties are of two types — (a) duties to yourself that are natural like taking bath, eating food, doing exercises etc., and secondly (b) duties which are imposed and are obligatory which we have accepted in relationship with others like duties towards our children.

2. *ARTHA*: Usually means wealth and money. We translate it here as barter or compensation — when certain acts are done and we are paid for it in exchange to a labour or service, like service in an office for which you get payment or salary.

3. *KAMA*: Generally taken as the sex enjoyment but it has a wider meaning. What about going for a picnic; going to a party to enjoy a pleasant and charming company, perfumes; ornaments etc. These all are thus part

of the process of the pursuit of pleasure. So, we say all actions for pleasure-quest through emotions or sex or whenever pleasure is sought, come under the category of kama.

4.*MOKSHA*: Older meaning is salvation or liberation. But in fact all actions which do not fall under the first three categories — not concerned with duty, not dependent upon material gain and not even for pleasure-quest, such actions generally come under moksha. Actions performed with the spirit of altruism, connected with the noble quality of self-sacrifice (selfless service), done with unselfish love which has a deep subconscious feeling of service, come under this category. "Unselfish love has enormous creative and therapeutic potentialities far greater than most people think," Sorokins says. Acts of this nature elevate us and bring us nearer to the spiritual life and that leads to moksha — the purpose of self-realization.

These motivations are sometimes correlated with each other or go in combination — a businessman may undertake a business deal combining a pleasure trip or a nurse working on salary may have a touch of moksha or may be in the case of a temple priest he may include all the four elements of motivation in the nature of his work. So, human actions may be prompted singly or in combination of these fourfold motivations. The important thing is the awareness and clarity of motivation, with understanding of WHAT YOU WANT and WHY YOU WANT. It is like fixing a centre of a circle, otherwise how else can you draw a circle? Most of us remain confused or undecided about motivation or there may be bifurcation of motivation by smaller objectives in life. Anytime the basic motivation is not strong or is disturbed, one will find the result proportionately unsatisfactory and this leaves the individual frustrated.

Remember, strong motivation (M) is based on value judgement (V) and then alone a proper attitude (A) is cultivated which finally determines the behaviour (B) pattern.

M —> V —> A —> B

While pleasure is legitimate, an addiction occasions contempt and loss of wealth besides causing physical and mental problems. Lust for money reduces a man to being an exploiter. Yoga holds that its aim is to direct the aspirant initially to hold the artha and kama activities in bonds by the practice of dharma and moksha. The main theme and content of Indian culture is integration and harmonization of the diverse aspects of life (fourfold purusharthas) through which we proceed towards ultimate realization of the inner divine nature.

Start this programme of thinking and acquire the habit of analysing your various actions and activities of the body.

14
GUIDELINES FOR SELF-IMPROVEMENT

14.1 3 A's: AWARENESS, ACCEPTANCE AND ADJUSTMENT

Much of the unhappiness in the world can be attributed to lack of understanding or wrong understanding with regard to a given situation. Things happen the way they have to happen and not necessarily as we would like them to happen. We have to develop self-awareness and the ability to put things in the proper perspective. Bhagawad Gita tells us that we are all bound by the inexorable law of 'Karma' which not only accounts for the inequality among the individual embodied souls but also clearly indicates that our life is not a mere accident but part of a 'Great Design' not comprehensible to us. *Karma* follows man like his shadow. Seen in this light, even sufferings and hardships acquire a new meaning and, far from being instruments of punishment, are meant to contribute to our growth and development. The moment we enter the precincts of this world we find ourselves not just individual entities but placed in relation to certain people and circumstances beyond our control. Initially, it is the family towards which we have certain obligatory duties which have to be accepted without resentment. As we grow older our area of interaction expands into ever-widening circles. The important thing to remember is that we are inseparable from others in our personal and social relationship and are constantly interacting with circumstances, favourable or otherwise. There are occasions when for no fault of ours we get ill-treatment from our near and dear ones, when in spite of our best efforts things go awry and we find oursevles beleaguered by seemingly insurmountable problems. All this is due to our *Prarabdha Karma* (actions done in the previous birth) from which there is no escape. We have to reap the fruits of our past actions, good or bad, and have to pay off according to our balance sheet. Whenever things go wrong we tend to blame the external circumstances or lack of proper opportunities or fate but disown our responsibility. We forget that the real trouble lies not with the external factors but with us who react to a particular situation in a particular way. The same external factors may affect different people differently. One may have an exaggerated notion of a problem and get upset easily while another may take things in his stride and can work positively to solve the problem. If an individual does not have the courage and the confidence to face a difficult situation, he will try to run away from it but that is nothing but self-deception. What is needed is patience and training of mind towards poise and equanimity so as to bring about a change in the habitual reaction pattern and develop the capacity to handle the situation in a constructive way. Have unflinching faith in God and rest assured that even though he may place you in a trying situation he will never test you beyond your capacity and will always give you guidance and strength throughout the period of travail. You have to learn to accept things as they happen, without getting agitated about them and patiently wait for the change to come. Everything in this world is in a state of flux, so change is bound to come. Every phase is transitory and will be superseded by another. Escapist tendency will not take you anywhere; you have to learn to accept the reality. Remember, the root cause of all our inner tension and turmoil is the intensity of our reaction. It can lead to a violent outburst or throw us into an abyss of depression. In either case, one loses the sense of discrimination and cannot see things objectively. Hence the need to develop self-awareness and to accept the inevitable.

Life demands adjustment if we are to live in harmony with ourselves and with our environment, whether at home or the place of work. Life is what we think. What is needed is clarity of thinking which may enable us to evaluate a given situation so that we can arrive at a correct judgement. We should look at the positive aspects of everything that happens from within and without. Through critical self-awareness we have to examine the validity of our value judgement which will ultimately determine whether a thing should be taken as good or bad. Personal adjustment involves a certain flexibility of outlook and a skill for better adaptability so that you feel at ease in any situation and can avoid extreme reactions. All that you need is proper self-direction and strong will-power to overcome negative emotions which manifest themselves in psychosomatic conditions. Our inner tension is reflected in external symptoms like sweating, hairpulling, shivering, stomach upset and so on. Our preoccupation with the external symptoms alone will not help since the real malady is in the mind, in our psyche. It is your behaviour and your reaction pattern which has to be changed. Yoga lays great emphasis on the inner personality which has to be properly moulded through constant practice. In order to follow the yoga way, we have to cultivate the right attitude towards others:

Friendliness towards those who are happy.
Compassion for those who are miserable.
Joyful participation with those who are virtuous.
Indifference towards those who are evil-minded.

This fourfold statement of Patanjali for better adjustment in life, practically covers the whole gamut of human relationships. If we follow this advice, we will be able to live in harmony with others and keep our mind calm and steady.

14.2 HOW WELL ADJUSTED YOU ARE: Questionnaire*

1. What is the last thing you do before going to bed?
   a) reading fiction/nothing special
   b) viewing TV/listening to music
   c) practice of Nishpanda Bhava; reading religious book or scriptures; practice of Bhavana (reflection); prayer
2. Night sleep
   a) disturbed or dreams
   b) fairly sound
   c) deep sleep
3. How much time do you spend in the morning walk, toilet, bath, newspaper reading and other household duties?
   a) more than 40 minutes
   b) 40 minutes
   c) 30 minutes.
4. How much time do you spend in your yoga routine practices?
   a) 10 minutes
   b) 20 minutes
   c) 30 minutes or more
5. In your breakfast do you have
   a) eggs and fried things etc.?
   b) toast, milk and fruits etc.?
   c) just a glass of milk, biscuit and fruits etc.?

* Courtesy: Mrs. G.Sahasi—Clinical Psychologist, Psychiatry Dept. AIIMS.

6. In job/office work, household work are you
   a) careless and unconcerned?
   b) average worker?
   c) conscientious and involved worker?
7. After lunch
   a) do you work immediately?
   b) take tea or coffee?
   c) relax?
8. After coming back from office what is the first thing that you do?
   a) sit with official work
   b) attend to wife, children and their needs
   c) conscious relaxation
9. In the evening hours do you generally like
   a) to visit friends/cinema/theatre/parties?
   b) outdoor games/club?
   c) to be with the family members and enjoy at home?
10. How much gap is there between dinner and sleep?
   a) half an hour
   b) one hour
   c) two hours
11. What normally guides your thoughts, tendencies and actions?
   a) convenience and comfort
   b) duty and convenience
   c) duty
12. When you notice untidiness or inefficiency which you could put right, what do you usually do?
   a) remain indifferent doing nothing?
   b) react with anger towards the person(s) responsible?
   c) correct the situation?
13. When you encounter obstacles in daily life, do you
   a) give up?
   b) go round or otherwise avoid them?
   c) try to remove them?
14. Do you get easily
   a) distracted?
   b) upset, excited and annoyed?
   c) absorbed in yourself or in what you do?
15. What is your disposition or natural temperament?
   a) easily vexed; moody
   b) average self-restraint

c) self-controlled

16. Feeling felt from life lived
    a) frustration/anxiety/worry
    b) neutral
    c) satisfaction and contentment

Scoring

The three alternatives a, b, c, in each question carry the score 1,2, and 3.

You are

POORLY ADJUSTED UP TO	27
MODERATELY ADJUSTED	28-37
WELL ADJUSTED	38-48

14.3 YOGA AND INNER TRANQUILLITY

In Yoga, the mind is understood in a more comprehensive way. It "forms a part of the *Chitta* — which represents all that is physical in man" (Shri Yogendra). The emphasis is laid on two important aspects of *Chitta*— PURITY AND QUIETUDE.

Yoga refers to the refining process at all levels of consciousness in case of man, as purification (shuddhi), as the sole pre-requisite and advocates an ideal synthesis and integration.

14.3.1 Asanas and Kriyas

The concept of purification is highly significant from health point of view and demands a conscious and planned endeavour to do away with unnatural and undesirable condition of the body-mind complex. The postural training programme as laid down in our Better Living courses with its many characteristics of exercises which are not too vigorous or strenuous, has a TOTAL approach. It therefore facilitates the correct interrelationship between psychosomatic and somatopsychic for the well being of human organism. To further help the yoga education of the body, there is a provision of KRIYAS — anti-toxic purificatory process (deha shuddhi) for different organs — keeping them in a healthy condition. Your mind then is free from bodily ill-health, discomfort and disease. In short, through asanas and *kriyas* and their hygienic effect on the Nervous system (Nadi Shuddhi) it is quite possible to influence even the mental processes and moral behaviour.

14.3.2 Breathing Process

There is an intimate connection between breathing and thought-waves. Steady inhalation and exhalation as advocated in the set of first four simplified Yogendra pranayamas induce calmness. The yogic method of harmonious and deep breathing brings about a sedative effect on the nerves and you achieve MENTAL EQUILIBRIUM. By correct understanding and use of pranayama, there is a gain in the energy content of the body and you also achieve certain stability of mind.

14.3.3 Yamaniyama

Ethical purity (Chitta-shuddhi) is the preliminary step and will help the individual to get rid of ignoble traits of his character. One has to develop pure and sincere love in the heart without any selfish claim and desire.

14.3.4 Conditioning and Psychosomatic Practices

To use one word for all such practices one can say they act as a QUIETENING PROCESS to make your mind CALM. The calmer we are, the less disturbed would be our nerves which will eventually result in better concentration and performance of work. Dexterity of action for efficiency and perfection whatever be your vocation in life, give you satisfaction and joy. Everything helps you to the fullest integration and expression of the human personality. Our conditioning process and psychosomatic practices of Yoni Mudra, Yogendra Nishpanda Bhava and Savasana can really give you a subjective experience of QUIETUDE or inner withdrawal. They destroy fatigue and calm the restless and agitated mind. Success in yoga fundamentally depends on uninterrupted and sustained practice and cultivation of a positive attitude of detachment and dispassion. It will then be easier for you to enter into Calm, Peaceful Inner Silence that goes deeper and stills thought and will. *Vritti nirodha* is the keynote. Patanjali defines yoga as the Control of mental modifications — *chitta vritti* — (The Thought waves of the Chitta).

Edward Bach, an eminent doctor says: "We must steadfastly practise PEACE, imagining our minds as a lake ever to be kept calm, without waves or even ripples to disturb its TRANQUILLITY, and gradually develop this state of PEACE until no event of life, no circumstance, no other personality is able, under any condition, to ruffle the surface of that lake or raise within, any feelings of irritability, depression or doubt."

14.4 HOW TO CARRY ON YOUR WORK
The Importance of Karma Yoga

> "Thy business is with the action only, never with its fruits; so let not the fruit of action be thy motive, nor be Thou to inaction attached."
>
> (from *Gita* II-47)

The above shloka which contains Lord Krishna's advice to Arjuna also offers the best guidelines in our day-to-day life.

Bhagawad Gita is a general treatise on yoga giving many definitions of and containing many terms associated with yoga practices. It contains many psychical observations and offers practical solutions to many of our day-to-day problems. The whole thing can be taken as a programme of wise counselling given by Lord Krishna to Arjuna whom he finds full of doubts and having acute neurotic symptoms leading to distress.

Symbolically, the battle of Kurukshetra is being fought within each one of us with all our inner conflicts, doubts and negative thoughts and like Arjuna, we are not willing to take up a challenge and we do not take our work in the spirit of karma yoga.

Activity is synonymous with life itself. Every individual in the world is created to engage himself in some activity at all levels and stages of his evolution. Howsoever one may try to run away from the world there is no escape from activity. Physical withdrawal into solitude will not help since the mind cannot be at rest. Moreover, abandonment of action leads us to a state of stupor and inertia which is a manifestation of the *Tamasic* element in us. In yoga sutra (Ch.I-30) the sage, Patanjali, describes the various obstacles, essentially psychosomatic in nature, which a practising yogi has to guard against. The first five of them like disease, dullness, doubt, carelessness and laziness are related to the *Tamasic* condition and take us away from action and thus from life itself.

Everybody, who is born in the world, brings with him a certain nature (Prakriti or Swabhava). It represents the aggregate of his innate tendencies from which he is inseparable. Its hold is so strong that it constantly propels a person, to act in a certain way. This inherent nature determines one's aptitude in life and takes him towards self-fulfilment. Since it is not possible to escape one's Prakriti, it is not possible to escape karma. The important thing to remember is that we should have the right ATTITUDE towards work and life. For a true karma yogi, karma itself is the yoga. One has to accept whatever comes in one's way and not consider any work superior or inferior. With one's limited vision and lack of perspective, one may not be able to correctly judge the righteousness or the unrighteousness of actions, and decide on the right priorities. Do your duties remembering that you are only an instrument in the hands of God who is the final arbiter of all actions. With this attitude, the ego will be transcended, all *karmas* will become equal in your eyes and everything that you do will be divinised. FREEDOM IN ACTION is possible only if one is able to free oneself from the expectation of results. *Karma* in itself is not a source of bondage, it is the thoughts about the outcome, successful or otherwise, which cause all the trouble, since the mind will constantly oscillate between the two opposite poles of success and defeat, delight or depression. There is no denying the fact that any karma that is performed is a means to achieve a specific end. We have to understand that there is no point in bothering about the results since every karma will inevitably bring its destined result. No one can escape the law of karmic results. It is a different matter, however, that the results may not be in accordance with our expectations. In spite of our best efforts, the outcome may be partial or even adverse since there are so many factors at work which are beyond our control. Things do not always happen the way we want them to happen. When we are engaged in our work we should keep in mind all the possibilities and try to exercise EQUANIMITY in the face of both success and failure. Preoccupation with the results can be a big distraction in the right performance of the work at hand. Yoga has been described in the Gita as "skill in action". To perform well, what is needed is total absorption in the activity of the moment, with the physical, mental and vital force acting in unison with a strong motivation to bring out the best in you. If a painter while painting is preoccupied with the thoughts of money or fame, a doctor while treating a serious case has his eye on the pocket, the performance will suffer since wholeheartedness towards the activity will be missing.

A true *karma* yogi combines deepest interest with perfect detachment. Every moment of activity is a moment of accomplishment, of joy, since his joy lies in the activity itself, not in the fruits of activity. When we do our work out of love, there is no expectation since love is an act of giving — giving our best, our whole self spontaneously. In such a moment our self does not exist, only the pursuit of love exists and we become what we do. We are absolutely free and yet absolutely absorbed.

WORKING FOR LOVE IS INDEED FREEDOM IN ACTION.

Remember

1. Engage yourself in your duty and work with a sense of total participation.
2. Do not consider any work superior or inferior.
3. Transcend the 'I'. Remember that you are not the doer but only an instrument of action.
4. Freedom from desire is the real freedom.
5. Live in the 'Now' in a dynamic way without burden of the past and consideration of the future.
6. Cultivate faith in a higher reality of The Absolute and function as a part of the larger process of life.

APPENDIX 1

12 BL Course (Basic) for Men and Women

Guide Table **40 Minutes a Day**

Sequ-ence	Yoga Posture		Yogendra Rhythm	Frequency (Rounds/Times)
1.	SUKHASANA or VAJRASANA	alter each day	Normal breathing	5 to 7 minutes
2.	TALASANA I,II,III VARS		INH RET EXH 3 : 6 : 3 SUS 3	4 times each variation
3.	KONASANA I VAR (Men) KONASANA II VAR (Women)		INH RET EXH 3 : 6 : 3	3 times alternate bending each side
4.	UTKATASANA (Men) NATAP RARTHANASANA (Women)		INH RET EXH 4 : 2 : 2 SUS INH EXH 4 : 2 : 2	6 times
5.	YOGA MUDRA in SUKHASANA	To start INH	EXH SUS INH 3 : 6 : 3	3 rounds
6.	VAKRASANA	To start first INH	EXH INH 3 : 3	5 times alternately each side
7.	BHUJANGASANA		INH RET EXH 3 : 6 : 3	5 times
8.	YOGENDRA PRANAYAMA No. 4 (Abdominal breathing) in lying-down position		Start with easy count to reach to a max of 8 seconds INH-EXH gradually	10 rounds
9.	SAVASANA		Normal breathing	7/10 minutes
10.	TRATAK i)Right shoulder gaze ii)Left shoulder gaze		Normal breathing; start with easy duration, to reach a max of two minutes gaze	3 times alternate each shoulder
11.	YOGENDRA PRANAYAMA No. 1 (in standing)		Start with easy counts to reach gradually 15 seconds of INH-EXH	10 rounds
12.	YOGENDRA NISPANDABHAVA		Normal breathing	10 minutes

N.B. * Inhalation: INH; Retention: RET; Exhalation:EXH; Suspension:SUS; Count to be maintained by mentally counting "ONE-THOUSAND ONE" which accounts for one second — verify with your watch and catch the rhythm.

* JALANETI(water snuffing) — Once or twice a week. More frequently if you suffer from a common cold, have a nasal block or sinusitis, etc.

APPENDIX 2

24 BL Course (General)

For Men

Guide Table **60 Minutes a Day**

Sequ-ence	Yoga Posture		Yogendra Rhythm	Frequency (Rounds/Times)
1.	SUKHASANA or VAJRASANA or PADMASANA	alter each day	Normal breathing	5 minutes
2.	TALASANA I,II,III VARS		INH RET EXH SUS 3 : 6 : 3 : 3	4 times each variation
3.	KONASANA I VAR		INH RET EXH 3 : 6 : 3	3 times alternate bending each side
4.	KONASANA III VAR		EXH SUSP INH 3 : 6 : 3	3 times alternate bending forward right and left toe
5.	UTKATASANAI or II VAR		INH RET EXH SUS 2 : 4 : 2 : 4 INH EXH 2 : 2	6 times
6.	HASTAPADAN-GUSTASANA I,II, III VARS		EXH INH 3 : 3 To start INH	3 times each variation with alternate leg
7.	CHAKRASANA I VAR		INH RET EXH INH 3 : 6 : 3 : 3	5 times
8.	KAPAL BHATI		Quick Oxygenation INH-EXH	4/6 cycles vigorously
9.	BHADRASANA (dynamic way)		INH RET EXH 3 : 10 : 2	4 times
10.	YOGA MUDRA in PADMASANA or SUKHASANA		EXH SUS INH 3 : 6 : 3	3 rounds
11.	ARDHAMATSYEN-DRASANA		To start INH EXH SUS INH 3 : 6	4 times alter twist or right and left
12.	JANUSIRASANA		To start INH EXH SUS INH 3 : 6 : 3	4 times with alternate leg
13.	PASCHIMOTTAN-ASANA (dynamic way)		To start INH EXH SUS INH 3 : 4 : 3	6 times
14.	BHUJANGASANA		INH RET EXH 3 : 6 : 3	5 times

15.	SHALABHASANA I & II VAR or DHANURASANA If difficult, prepare yourself by doing NAUKASANA Type (raising both legs and thorax)	EXH SUSP INH 3 : 6 : 3 INH RET EXH 3 : 6 : 3	4 times 4 times
16.	PAVANMUKT-ASANA (Ekapada) I VAR or (DWIPADA) — II VAR	To start INH EXH SUS INH 2 : 4 : 2 "	4 times alternately with each leg — I VAR or with both the legs
17.	ARDHSARVANGASANA or VIPARITAKARANI or SARVANGASANA	EXH-STATIC PAUSE 4 2 Mints: INH 4 in static pause slow rhythmic breathing — gradually increase the pause to 2 mnts.	Once only
18.	HALASANA	Normal slow rhythmic breating	Once only 1 mnt
19.	SAVASANA	Normal breathing	5 minutes
20.	TRATAK: i) right shoulder gaze — alter each day ii) left shoulder gaze or iii) Tip of the nose — alter each day iv) space between eyebrows	Normal breathing "	Do once if you have reached a gaze of 2 mins. duration, other wise do 3 times each type of Tratak "
21.	Y. PRANAYAMA No.2 (in standing)	Starting with easy count to reach gradually INH-EXH	10 rounds 10 seconds 10 rounds
22.	Y.PARANAYAMA No. 4 (in sitting)	increase to 8 seconds	
	or		
	Y.PRANAYAMA No. 5 (SUNYAKA)	Begin with 5 seconds SUSP gradually increase to 20/30 seconds	10 rounds with pause of normal breathing after each round
23.	YOGA ALTERNATE BREATHING	3 breaths/minute or 2 breaths/minute	4 rounds
	or		
	YOGIC COMPLETE BREATH	INH = EXH slow normal breathing	5 rounds 10 minutes
24.	YOGENDRA NISHPANDABHAVA	Normal breathing	10 minutes

APPENDIX 3

24 BL Course (General)
For Women

Guide Table **40 Minutes a Day**

Sequ-ence	**Yoga Posture**	**Yogendra Rhythm**	**Frequency (Rounds/Times)**
1.	SUKHASANA or VAJRASANA or PADMASANA — alter each day	Normal breathing	5 min.
2.	EPADASANA	Normal breathing	3 times with each leg. Gradually increase the static pause to 1 minute
3.	YASHTIKASANA or TALASANA I,II,II, VARS	INH RET EXH SUS 3 : 6 : 3 : 3	4 times each variation
4.	KONASANA II VAR	INH RET EXH 3 : 6 : 3	3 times alternate bending forward
5.	KONASANA III VAR	EXH SUS INH 3 : 6 : 3	3 times alternate bending forward right and left toe
6.	TRIKONASANA or HASTAPADASANA	EXH SUS INH 3 : 6 : 3	5 times
7.	NATA PRARTHANASANA	INH RET EXH 2 : 4 : 2 SUS INH EXH 4 : 2 : 2	6 times
8.	HASTAPADANGUSTASANA I,II,III VARS	EXH INH 3 : 3	3 times each variation with alternate leg
9.	USTRASANA	INH RET EXH 3 : 6 : 3	5 times
10.	KAPAL BHATI	Quick Oxygenation INH-EXH	4/6 cycles vigorously
11.	PARVATASANA I,II,III YAR	INH RET EXH 3: 6: 3	3 times each variation
12.	YOGA MUDRA in Padmasana or Sukhasana	EXH SUS INH 3 : 6 : 3	3 rounds
13.	PASCHIMOTTANASANA (dynamic way)	EXH SUS INH 3 : 4 : 3 To start INH	6 times To start INH
	or		
	JANUSIRASANA	EXH SUSP INH 3 : 6 : 3 To start with INH	4 times with alternate leg
14.	ARDHAMATSYENDRASANA	EXH SUS INH 3 : 6 : 3	4 times alternate twist on right and left 3 times.

15.	MATSYASANA	INH RET EXH 3 : 6 : 3	Repeat three times alternately maintain the pose for one or two minutes with normal breathing
16.	PARYANKASANA or If difficult, try SUPTA VAJRASANA Type	INH RET EXH 4 : 6 : 3	5 times (gradually increase the static pause to a max of 2 1/2 min with slow rhythmic breathing and do it only once)
17.	BHUJANGASANA or	To start with INH INH RET EXH 3 : 6 : 3	5 times
	SHALABHASANA I,II VAR or	EXH SUSP INH 3 : 6 : 3	4 times
	DHANURASANA	INH RET EXH 3 : 6 : 3	4 times
18.	VIPARITAKARANI	EXH INH 4:1/2 mnt to 4 2 mnts: (in static pause, slow rhythmic breathing)	only once
19.	HALASANA	Normal slow rhythmic breathing	Once only for 1 mnt
20.	SAVASANA	Normal breathing	5 minutes
21.	TRATAK: i)right shoulder gaze ii)left shoulder gaze or alter iii)tip of the nose or each iv)space between the day eyebrows	Normal breathing	Do once if you have reached a gaze of 2 mins. otherwise do 3 times each type of Tratak
22.	Y.PRANAYAMA No.I or YOGIC COMPLETE BREATH	Starting with easy count gradually increase to 14 seconds INH-EXH	10 rounds
23.	Y.PRANAYAMA No. 2 (in standing) and	Starting with easy count gradually	10 rounds
	Y.PRANAYAMA No. 4 (in sitting or lying down)	increase to 10 sec INH-EXH	10 rounds
24.	YONI MUDRA or YOGENDRA alter NISHPANDA BHAVA each or MAKARASANA day	Normal breathing	10 minutes each

APPENDIX 4

TABLE*

"Desirable" Body Weight in Adults

Height (with shoes, 1-inch heels)		**Average weight for "medium" frame**			
		Men		**Women**	
Feet	**Inches**	**Lbs**	**Kgs**	**Lbs**	**Kgs**
4	10	...	...	102	46
4	11	...	...	104	47
5	0	...	...	107	49
5	1	...	...	110	50
5	2	124	56	113	51
5	3	127	58	116	53
5	4	130	59	120	55
5	5	133	60	123	56
5	6	137	62	128	58
5	7	140	64	132	60
5	8	145	66	136	62
5	9	149	68	140	64
5	10	153	70	144	65
5	11	158	72	148	67
6	0	162	74	152	69
6	1	167	76	...	...
6	2	171	78	...	...
6	3	176	80	...	...
6	4	181	82	...	...

After the age of 40 years, it is best to keep the weight slightly below the average as it helps to lighten the burden on the heart, kidneys and other vital organs.

**Heart Care*, April-June 1971.

SOME ESPECIALLY BENEFICIAL ASANAS FOR WOMEN

- IN STANDING POSITION
  - EKPADASANA
  - TALASANA/YASHTIKASANA
  - KONASANA II VR.
  - TRIKONASANA
  - USTARASANA
- IN SITTING POSITION
  - PARVATASANA
  - YOGA MUDRA
  - ARDHAMATSYENDRASANA
- IN LYING-DOWN POSITION
  - MATSYASANA
  - BHUJANGASANA
  - PARYANKASANA
  - HALASANA
- HEAD-LOW POSITION
  - VIPARITKARANI

BIBLIOGRAPHY

Heal Thyself, Bach Edward, 1957, Rochford, The C.W. Daniel Company Ltd.

Commense Vegetarianism, Benjamin Harry, 1972, Northants, Thorsons Publishers Limited.

Abnormal Psychology and Modern Life, Coleman James, 1956, Scott, Foresman & Company.

About Vegetarian Diet, Dangayach K.B., Vol.XXI, No. 1, Aug. 1975, Bombay, Journal of the Yoga Institute.

Hatha Yoga, Ramacharaka Yogi, Asian Reprint, 1977, Bombay, D.B. Taraporevala Sons & Co., (P) Ltd.

Practical Nature-Cure, Sharma, K. Lakshmana, 1978 (12th Ed.), Pudukottai, The Nature-Cure Publishing House.

Yoga against Spinal Pain, Sharma, Pandit Shiv, 1971, Delhi-Bombay-Calcutta - Madras, B.I. Publications.

Food Remedies, Singh S.J.,1947, Lucknow, The All India Nature Cure Association.

Self-Improvement, The Yoga Sadhakas, 1980, Bombay, The Yoga Institute.

Pranayama Made Easy, The Yoga Sadhakas, 1981, Bombay, The Yoga Institute, Yogendra Publications.

Yoga Hygiene Simplified, Shri Yogendra, 1975, Bombay, The Yoga Institute.

Yoga Essays, Shri Yogendra, 1973, Bombay, The Yoga Institute.

Hatha Yoga Simplified, Shri Yogendra, 1975, Bombay, The Yoga Institute.

Guide To A Fuller Life, The Yoga Institute, 1986, Bombay, Yogendra Publications.

Yoga Physical Education For Women, Yogendra Sitadevi, 1981, Bombay, Yogendra Publications Fund.

Guide to Yoga Meditation, Shri Yogendra, 1983, Bombay Yogendra Publication Fund.

The Philosophy of Action, Mangalvedkar, 1923, Madras, B.G. Tilka's Githa Rahasya, The Indian Literature Publisher.

Physiological Psychology, Wenger M.A., Jones F.N., Jones, M.H. 1956, New York, University of California, Los Angeles.

Yoga, Wood Ernest, reprinted 1968, A Pelican Original-Penguin Book.
Melbourne High Blood Pressure, Victoria 3000, Prepared and Produced by the Editorial Committee of Science of Life Books.

Periodicals

Reducing Tensions, page 150, Sequeira H, Vol. XXV, No. 9, April 1980, Bombay, Journal of the Yoga Institute.
Stability of Mind, page 6, Sequeira, Vol. XXIV No. 7, February 1984, Bombay, Journal of the Yoga Institute.
Tranquil State of Mind of the Gita, page 165, Vol. XX,No.11, June 1975, Bombay, Journal of the Yoga Institute.
How to Carry on Your Work, page 145, Yogendra Jayadeva, Vol. XXI, No. 10, May 1975, Bombay, Journal of the Yoga Institute.
April June 1971 issue, Heart Care, Bombay, Published by Commerce (1935) Ltd. on behalf of the Society for Prevention of Heart Disease and Rehabilitation.